T0211269

Clinical Optics Primer for Ophthalmic Medical Personnel

A Guide to Laws, Formulae, Calculations, and Clinical Applications

Clinical Optics Primer for Ophthalmic Medical Personnel

A Guide to Laws, Formulae, Calculations, and Clinical Applications

Aaron V. Shukla, PhD, COMT
Associate Professor and Program Director
Ophthalmic Technician Program
St. Catherine University
Minneapolis, MN

Director of Education
Eye Care Associates, P.A.
Minneapolis, MN

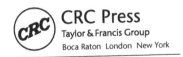

CRC Press
Taylor & Francis Group
Boca Raton London New York

CRC Press is an imprint of the
Taylor & Francis Group, an **informa** business

Cover photographs by Aaron V. Shukla.

First published 2009 by SLACK Incorporated

Published 2024 by CRC Press
2385 NW Executive Center Drive, Suite 320, Boca Raton FL 33431

and by CRC Press
4 Park Square, Milton Park, Abingdon, Oxon, OX14 4RN

CRC Press is an imprint of Taylor & Francis Group, LLC

Visit the Taylor & Francis Web site at
http://www.taylorandfrancis.com

and the CRC Press Web site at
http://www.crcpress.com

Library of Congress Cataloging-in-Publication Data

Clinical optics primer for ophthalmic medical personnel : a guide to laws, formulae, calculations, and clinical applications / Aaron V. Shukla.
　　p. ; cm.
Includes bibliographical references and index.
ISBN 978-1-55642-899-9 (alk. paper)
1. Physiological optics. 2. Ophthalmic assistants. I. Title.
[DNLM: 1. Refractive Errors--diagnosis--Handbooks. 2. Contact Lenses--Handbooks. 3. Eyeglasses--Handbooks. 4. Ophthalmic Assistants--Handbooks. 5. Ophthalmology--methods--Handbooks. 6. Vision Disorders--Handbooks. WW 39 S562c 2009]
QP475.S555 2009
612.8'4--dc22

2008046243

ISBN: 9781556428999 (pbk)
ISBN: 9781003523109 (ebk)

DOI: 10.1201/9781003523109

Dedication

To
Arielle and Jordana

My daughters,
My best friends,
My greatest fans.
A long time ago,
We grew up together,
They, in their years,
I, in my profession.

Contents

SECTION I. IMPORTANT LAWS OF OPTICS AND THEIR CLINICAL APPLICATIONS

SECTION II. IMPORTANT FORMULAE AND CONSTANTS IN OPTICS AND THEIR CLINICAL APPLICATIONS

Acknowledgments

Many rungs make a ladder, and many people are responsible for making this book possible, and I owe thanks and gratitude to them.

My editors at SLACK Incorporated for noticing a worthy idea and making it possible, and then for putting up with my idiosyncrasies.

My professional colleagues who willingly reviewed portions of the book (in alphabetical order):

Debra J. Baker, MA, COMT
John L. Baker, OD
Larry Bovard, COT
Shawn L. Brown, CO, COMT
Susan K. Brummett, COMT
C. Sue Campbell, COMT
Debra B. Clarke, COT
Deborah Diggins, COMT
Nora J. Gould, COMT
Dinesh Goyal, MD
Suzanne J. Hansen, COMT
Richard A. Harper, MD
Barbara Harris, PA, COA
Beth Koch, COT
Paul M. Larson, COMT, COE
Jo A. Legacki, COMT
Andrew Lima, COA
Eva Lindahl, COMT
Natalie Loyacano, COMT, ROUB, OCS
Carol J. Pollack-Rundle, COMT
Christine Romero, COT
Lisa Rovick, CO, COMT
Mary K. Smit, COT
Karen Susco, COMT
P. Keith Thompson, MD
Duanne Van Camp, COT
Shirley Weiss, COMT
Lori J. Williams, COMT
Michelle Willis, COMT
Andy Winters, COMT
Ken Woodworth, COMT, COE

Dinesh K. Goyal, MD, for providing me with valuable clinical education, discussions, encouragement, and camaraderie during a busy ophthalmology practice, and for writing a foreword for this book.

About the Author

Aaron Shukla was born and raised in Lucknow, India, a state capital in the north Indian state of Uttar Pradesh. With forebears in medicine, he was keen on a medical career. As an undergraduate in Lucknow University, he also became interested in geology, mineralogy, and crystallography, and thus pursued both majors.

He arrived in the United States in 1974, earning a master's degree in geology from Princeton University in New Jersey, and a doctorate in 1980 from Rensselaer Polytechnic Institute in New York State. Subsequently, he worked as a senior geologist for Texaco in Houston, TX. While there, his work interests included geochemistry, mineralogy, and using polarized light and electron beams to interpret changes in petroleum rocks and sediments that produce pore spaces in which oil and gas can accumulate. He was particularly interested in using optics and light phenomena for mineralogy.

But, the embers of medical interests continued to smolder!

In 1996, he graduated with honors from Portland Community College, Portland, OR, earning an associate of applied science degree in ophthalmic medical technology. From there he started on the long road to acquiring experiences and expertise as a COT, then as a COMT, in clinic and surgery. Of particular interest were optics, strabismus, visual fields, neuro-ophthalmology, and pediatric ophthalmology.

In 2000, Dr. Shukla joined the University of Arkansas for Medical Sciences (UAMS), Little Rock, AR. As an assistant professor at UAMS, he was the founding chairman of the Department of Ophthalmic Technologies and its technologist-level education program for the College of Health Related Professions and The Harvey and Bernice Jones Eye Institute of the Department of Ophthalmology, School of Medicine. The technologist program earned its initial accreditation in 2004 and is continuing with great success. The graduates of that program became the first COMTs in Arkansas.

Successes in Arkansas brought opportunities, and in 2004, Dr. Shukla joined the Joint Commission on Allied Health Personnel in Ophthalmology (JCAHPO) as its founding director of program and services. At JCAHPO, he was instrumental in developing the Learning Systems, the interactive DVD for ophthalmic medical personnel (OMP) interested in learning keratometry, tonometry, lensometry, visual fields, ocular motility, retinoscopy, and refinement. These modules are also of critical use in preparing for JCAHPO's COT Skill Test for certification.

In 2005, he joined Eye Care Associates, P.A., Minneapolis, MN, as its director of education, while also providing services as a COMT.

In 2006, Dr. Shukla joined St. Catherine University as an associate professor and founding program director of the Ophthalmic Technician Program—a technician-level education program.

Dr. Shukla has been a volunteer faculty member for JCAHPO and Association of Technical Personnel in Ophthalmology (ATPO) since 1996, giving lectures and workshops at annual and regional meetings, and he has published articles on optics, clinical work, and various tests and procedures. He continues to be active with JCAHPO and ATPO, and was elected ATPO's vice president in 2007. He will assume responsibilities as its president in 2009, and immediate past president in 2010.

Preface

Clinical applications, success in certification examinations, and helping to build a relevant knowledge base to achieve these goals is the standard that a book such as this one must meet.

In the author's experience, ophthalmic medical personnel (OMP), which includes COAs, COTs, and COMTs, are generally united in their intense dislike of ophthalmic optics. This is mystifying because success in certification examinations and excellence in clinical work require a good comprehension of this subject. Most measurements and procedures in an eye clinic and ophthalmic surgery are performed with the aim of improving the optics of the human eye. Still, malaise prevails!

Many books currently available for ophthalmic optics provide explanations of the concepts of light and optics, including laws and formulae governing light and its various phenomena important for understanding the optimal working of the human eye. However, those explanations do not provide details that can be easily understood by OMP, nor do those books provide enough examples of optical calculations or sufficiently extensive examples of clinical applications. Perhaps this is why discussions on ophthalmic optics draw wide yawns.

In the author's experience, the greatest problem faced by OMP is the inability to readily recall important laws, as well as the inability to readily calculate simple but important parameters such as focal length and diopters. There also appears to be a wide chasm between the theory of ophthalmic optics and direct clinical applications. Oddly enough, these tendencies increase with greater experience.

The aim of this book is to present laws, formulae, basic optical mathematics, and calculations in a simple and concise way, while also providing many examples of simple calculations and extensive examples of clinical applications, all in one place. Thus, this book will make reviewing the material much easier, and it will also serve as a ready reference. The book will also complement existing texts on ophthalmic optics.

I have used all of the concepts outlined in this book during my professional career, and with great success. Feedback from patients and ophthalmologists has been overwhelmingly positive. My hope is that this book will go a long way toward lifting the veil of anxiety and uncertainty for OMP when they perform ophthalmic tests and measurements.

Foreword

The practice of medicine has evolved into a more team-oriented approach in recent years. As populations grow and our understanding of human medicine becomes increasingly complex, we have come to rely on various levels of healthcare personnel to deliver good patient care. Visiting the doctor involves examination by multiple professionals, all of whom must be well trained in their respective fields.

Ophthalmologists rely heavily on skilled COAs, COTs, and COMTs to conduct many of the key components of an eye examination. Almost any portion of this examination can be related to the clinical applications of optics. Perhaps one of the most important, yet overlooked, uses of clinical optics occurs when measuring refractive errors of patients. Technical staff must be able to integrate the knowledge of optical properties of the human eye in its different states with that of light, lenses, and instrumentation to accurately measure for spectacle, contact, and even intraocular lenses. A good technician is one who can accurately determine possible imperfections in the optical system of the human eye, and help lead to an effective resolution.

In this *Clinical Optics Primer for Ophthalmic Medical Personnel*, Dr. Aaron Shukla has taken a relatively difficult and often feared subject, and turned it into one that can be easily understood and applied. Dr. Shukla has not only provided us with the tools of optics, but he has clearly and concisely demonstrated their use in numerous clinical case examples. Key formulae and facts are presented in an easy-to-follow tabular format, and the illustrations are his original ones. Learning objectives, summary notes, and review questions in each chapter help to solidify the reader's understanding of the most salient points. Ophthalmic assistants, technicians, and technologists will be able to quickly acquire the knowledge and immediately implement it into their everyday practice. This book will also act as an excellent study guide in preparation for certification examinations.

We, as health care professionals, share a commitment to deliver the best possible ophthalmic care to our patients. *Clinical Optics Primer for Ophthalmic Medical Personnel* by Dr. Aaron Shukla will help technical staff and physicians alike in achieving this goal. This book is uniquely comprehensive without the drudgery commonly associated with optics. It can be read and re-read by all students of ophthalmology as an introduction to, review of, and reference to optics.

Dinesh K. Goyal, MD
Eye Care Associates, P.A.
Minneapolis, MN

Introduction

A resident physician training to become an ophthalmologist once remarked to me, in an unusual moment of fascination with optics, that everything we do in diagnosing and treating ocular disorders and conditions is aimed at improving the optics of the eye. How true!

The purpose of the human eye is to produce the sharpest possible image on the fovea. Therefore, better visual acuity simply means that a person is able to perceive smaller and smaller images. To have good visual acuity, three things have to happen:

1. A sharp image must be produced.

2. The sharp image must be transmitted to the visual cortex.

3. The visual cortex must process the sharp image.

Any interruption in this process will result in decreased visual acuity.

In optics, we deal with how light is refracted into the eye, and reflected from the eye, in order to produce useful images. The lenses and mirrors used to produce the most useful images are a measurement of the refractive states of the eye.

This book is designed for use by ophthalmic medical personnel (OMP) who are involved with measuring refractive errors, evaluating glasses and contact lenses, and using various ophthalmic instruments that utilize lenses and mirrors.

The book is written in an easy, conversational style and is ideally suited for OMP who might not have a strong background in the physics of light and optics.

The book introduces important phenomena used every day in ophthalmic tests, measurements, and procedures, and the material in each chapter briefly, but comprehensively, explains important points. Each chapter starts with a description, learning objectives, and key points, then continues with explaining the subject matter while including examples of calculations and clinical applications, and concludes with review questions that can be answered by considering material presented in the chapter.

To assist readers, the first two chapters are devoted to metric units of measurements and basic mathematics for optics—all of which are necessary for clinical applications.

Finally, the book also includes references at the end of some chapters for those OMP who might wish to further investigate physical, geometric, and clinical (physiologic) optics.

SECTION I

IMPORTANT LAWS OF OPTICS AND THEIR CLINICAL APPLICATIONS

1

Metric System

Prefixes, Values, and Units of Measurement

The system for measurements in ophthalmic and other medical applications is the *metric system*, which is summarized in Table 1-1.

Table 1-1[1]

Prefixes and Values		Unit of Measure		
Prefix	**Value**	**Volume**	**Weight**	**Length**
Kilo-	1000 times (10^3) of BU		kilogram (kg)	Kilometer (km)
	Basic Unit (BU)	**liter (L)**	**gram (g)**	**meter (m)**
Deci-	$\frac{1}{10}$ or 0.1 times (10^{-1}) BU	deciliter (dL)[2]		
Centi-	$\frac{1}{100}$ or 0.01 times (10^{-2}) BU			centimeter (cm)
Milli-	$\frac{1}{1000}$ or 0.001 times (10^{-3}) BU	milliliter (mL)	milligram (mg)	millimeter (mm)

[1]Only commonly used prefixes and units of measurement are included. Standard texts may be consulted for additional prefixes and units of measurement.

[2]Used to document blood glucose (eg, 130 mg/dL).

CONVERTING UNITS OF MEASUREMENT

Ophthalmic calculations frequently require converting one unit of measurement into another (eg, m into cm, kg into mg). Such conversions may be easily accomplished by either multiplying or dividing by units of "10," (10, 100, 1000, etc). Table 1-2 lists commonly used conversions.

Table 1-2

To Convert This	To This...	Do This:
kilo-	BU (L, g, m)	Multiply by 1000
	deci-	Multiply by 10,000
	centi-	Multiply by 100,000
	milli-	Multiply by 1,000,000
Basic Unit (BU)	centi-	Multiply by 100
	milli-	Multiply by 1000
centi-	BU	Divide by 100
	deci-	Divide by 10
	milli-	Multiply by 10
milli-	kilo-	Divide by 1,000,000
	BU	Divide by 1000
	deci-	Divide by 100

EXAMPLE 1

A focal length of 2 m may also be stated in cm or mm:

For cm: Multiply m by 100 = 2 x 100 = 200 cm
For mm: Multiply m by 1000 = 2 x 1000 = 2000 mm

Example 2

The Humphrey Field Analyzer (Carl Zeiss Meditec, Dublin, CA) bowl has a radius of 30 cm, which may also be stated in m or mm:

For m: Divide cm by 100 $=$ $\frac{30}{100}$ $=$ 0.3 m

For mm: Multiply cm by 10 $=$ 30 x 10 $=$ 300 mm

Review Questions

1. A blood glucose reading of 130 mg/dL may also be stated as:
    a. 1300 mg/mL
    b. 13,000 mg/mL
    c. 13 mg/L
    d. 1.3 mg/L

2. 5 mL of fluorescein sodium may also be stated as:
    a. 5 dL
    b. 50 L
    c. 0.05 dL
    d. 500 L

3. A total intake of 4 tablets of amoxicillin, each 500 mg, may also be stated as:
    a. 2 g
    b. 1 g
    c. 0.01 mg
    d. 20 mg

4. A focal length of 50 cm may also be stated as:
    a. 0.5 m
    b. 5 m
    c. 0.5 mm
    d. 50 mm

5. Compared to a focal length of 1000 mm, a focal length of 1 m is:
    a. greater
    b. the same
    c. less
    d. variable

2

Basic Optical Math

Learning Objectives

Upon completion of this chapter, the reader should be able to:

o   rearrange basic optical equations.
o   perform basic optical calculations.

Key Points

o   Equations and variables.
o   Moving variables in an equation.
o   Calculate speed of light and refractive index; power of lenses, prisms, mirrors, and curved refractive surfaces; vergence; magnification by lenses; spherical equivalent; accommodation; decentration and induced prism; and base curves of spectacle and contact lenses.

Equations and Variables

Many measurements and procedures performed by ophthalmic medical personnel (OMP) involve calculations using *equations*, in which *variables* (quantities and units that can vary) on one side of the equation equal the variables on the other side, as shown below:

1 or more variables = 1 or more variables

eg,   Speed of light = (wavelength) x (frequency)

In ophthalmology, units associated with variables are expressed using the metric system for volume, weight, and length. An important rule to observe is that units used for variables must be expressed in the manner specified in the formula being used.

For example, an important rule in ophthalmology is *Prentice's Rule*, which specifies that the unit for *optical center displacement* must be expressed in cm when using the formula. However, the decentration is typically measured in mm, which must be converted to cm before the equation may be used. If this is not done, the calculated answer will be incorrect.

BASIC MATH FOR REARRANGING EQUATIONS

In many ophthalmic calculations, the basic equation must be rearranged in order to calculate the missing variable. Basic equations may include adding, subtracting, dividing, or multiplying variables, and specific rules must be followed to rearrange such equations.

Please see Basic Optical Math ahead for details on the variables used below:

EQUATIONS INVOLVING ADDING

$$\text{Vergence equation: } U + P = V$$

To calculate U, move P to the other side and change its sign:
$$U = V - P$$
To calculate P, move U to the other side and change its sign:
$$P = V - U$$

EQUATIONS INVOLVING SUBTRACTING

$$\text{Refractive index: } 0.336 = n - 1.000$$

To calculate n, move –1.000 to the other side, and change its sign:
$$n = 1 + 0.336 = 1.336$$

EQUATIONS INVOLVING DIVIDING

$$\text{Focal length: } f_{(m)} = \frac{1}{D}$$

To calculate D, switch its position with $f_{(m)}$:
$$D = \frac{1}{f_{(m)}}$$

EQUATIONS INVOLVING MULTIPLYING

$$\text{Induced prism}_{(PD \text{ or } \Delta)} = \text{Lens power}_{(D)} \times \text{OC displacement}_{(cm)}$$

To calculate Lens power$_{(D)}$, move the OC displacement$_{(cm)}$ to the other side and to the bottom, making it a denominator:

$$\frac{\text{Induced prism}_{(PD \text{ or } \Delta)}}{\text{OC displacement}_{(cm)}} = \text{Lens power}_{(D)}$$

To calculate OC displacement$_{(cm)}$, move the Lens power$_{(D)}$ to the other side and to the bottom, making it a denominator:

$$\frac{\text{Induced prism}_{(PD\ or\ \Delta)}}{\text{Lens power}_{(D)}} = \text{OC displacement}_{(cm)}$$

Basic Optical Math

Basic optical math calculations useful for OMP include the following parameters:
1. Speed of light and refractive index
2. Focal length and the power of lenses
3. Vergence equation
4. Magnification by lenses
5. Prism power
6. Power of mirrors
7. Coniod of Sturm and spherical equivalent
8. Refracting power of a curved surface
9. Base curve of spectacle lenses
10. Base curve of contact lenses
11. Amplitude of Accommodation
12. Prentice's rule, decentration, and induced prism

Basic optical math calculations for these parameters are described below.

Speed of Light and Refractive Index

Please see Chapter 4 for additional details.

Refractive Index (RI) is a ratio:

$$RI = \frac{\text{Speed of light in a vacuum}}{\text{Speed of light in a medium}} = \frac{3 \times 10^{10}\ \text{cm per sec}^*}{\text{Speed of light in a medium}}$$

Note: Some references state "air" instead of "vacuum," but technically it should be "vacuum."

*Non-metric units may also be used (eg, 186,000 miles/sec instead of 3×10^{10} cm/sec).

The speed of light in a medium can also be calculated by switching its position with the RI:

$$\text{Speed of light in a medium} = \frac{3 \times 10^{10}\ \text{cm per sec}^*}{RI}$$

*Non-metric units may also be used (eg, 186,000 miles/sec instead of 3×10^{10} cm/sec).

Example 1

What is the RI of a transparent medium in which light travels at a speed of 0.3×10^{10} cm/sec?

$$RI = \frac{3 \times 10^{10}\ \text{cm per sec}}{\text{Speed of light in a medium}}$$

$$RI = \frac{3 \times 10^{10}}{0.3 \times 10^{10}}$$

$$RI = \frac{3}{0.3} \times \frac{10^{10}}{10^{10}}$$

$$RI = \frac{3}{0.3} \times 1$$

$$RI = \frac{3}{0.3}$$

$$RI = \frac{30}{3}$$

$$RI = 10$$

Example 2

What is the speed of light in a normal tear film? (RI of tears is 1.336.)

$$\text{Speed of light in a medium} = \frac{3 \times 10^{10} \text{ cm per sec}}{RI}$$

$$\text{Speed of light in tears} = \frac{3 \times 10^{10} \text{ cm per sec}}{1.336}$$

$$\text{Speed of light in tears} = \frac{3}{1.336} \times 10^{10} \text{ cm/sec}$$

$$\text{Speed of light in tears} = 2.24 \times 10^{10} \text{ cm/sec}$$

Thus, light slows down by approximately 25% in the tear film as compared to a vacuum.

Since the RI of aqueous and vitreous are the same as tears, the speed of light and the percentage at which it slows down in aqueous and vitreous is the same as it is in tears.

Focal Length and the Power of Lenses

Please see Chapter 10 for additional details.

The power of plus and minus lenses, both spherical and cylindrical, is expressed in diopters (D), which is inversely related to focal length (f):

$$P_{(D)} = \frac{1}{f_{(m)}}$$

f may also be calculated by switching its position with P:

$$f_{(m)} = \frac{1}{P_{(D)}}$$

Example 3

Calculate the power of a lens whose f is 0.3 m.

$$P_{(D)} = \frac{1}{f_{(m)}}$$

$$P_{(D)} = \frac{1}{0.3}$$

$$P_{(D)} = \frac{10}{3}$$

$$P_{(D)} = 3.33 \text{ D}$$

Note: The distance from the corneal plane to the fixation light in a Goldmann perimeter and Humphrey Field Analyzer is 30 cm. For this reason, the basic power of a plus lens required for testing the visual field of presbyopes is +3.25 D (the value, 3.33 D, rounded off to the closest lower quarter). The actual lens used is obtained by considering +3.25 along with the refractive error and accommodative amplitude of the patient.

Example 4

Calculate f for a lens whose power is 2.75 D.

$$f_{(m)} = \frac{1}{P_{(D)}}$$

$$f_{(m)} = \frac{1}{2.75}$$

$$f_{(m)} = 0.36 \text{ m}$$

$$f_{(m)} = 36.4 \text{ cm}$$

Note: This is why the power of a reading add for pseudophakes is typically +2.75 D for a reading distance of approximately 36 cm. More plus power will be required to hold reading material closer, whereas less plus power will be required to hold it farther.

Vergence Equation

Please see Chapter 11 for additional details.

The powers of lenses and object-image relationships can be calculated more easily using the vergence equation:

$$U + P = V$$

Where:

U = object vergence (in D) = $\frac{1}{u}$ (u is the object distance in m)

P = lens power (in D)   = $\frac{1}{f}$ (f is the focal length in m)

V = image vergence (in D) = $\frac{1}{v}$ (v is the image distance in m)

Thus, vergence (in D) is simply the inverse of distance (object, focal, or image) in m.

Note: Since all light rays are divergent, a minus sign is assigned to object vergence in all calculations involving single lenses, thus making the vergence equation $-U + P = V$. In an array of multiple lenses, however, U may be plus or minus depending on the location of the object. Please see Chapter 12 for more details.

Example 5

Calculate the image vergence and image location for an object held 0.075 m in front of a +90 D lens. (NOTE: 1 m = 100 cm = 1000 mm.)

Object vergence in D (U) = $\frac{1}{u}$ (u is the object distance in m)

$$U = \frac{1}{0.075} = 13.3 \text{ D}$$

Image vergence (V) may now be calculated. Note that a minus sign is used for U in this example. If a proper algebraic sign is not assigned, the calculated value will be incorrect. Assigning algebraic signs is discussed in Chapter 11.

$$V = U + P$$
$$V = -(+13.3) + (+90)$$
$$V = -13.3 + 90$$
$$V = +76.7 \text{ D}$$

The plus sign in front of 76.7 D indicates that the image forms on the other side of the lens from the object. See Chapter 10 for details.

Image vergence, V, (+76.7 D) may be converted to image distance (image location):

Image distance in m $(v) = \dfrac{1}{V}$

$$v = \dfrac{1}{76.7}$$
$$v = 0.013 \text{ m}$$
$$v = 1.3 \text{ cm}$$

This is the reason that, during a dilated fundus examination, a +90 D lens is held approximately 5 cm from the eye, and the slit lamp beam is focused at approximately 1.3 cm from the +90 D lens in order to observe the fundus image.

Magnification by Lenses

Please see Chapter 13 for additional details.

Magnification may be determined by comparing the image distance to the object distance:

$$\text{Magnification} = \frac{\text{Image distance}}{\text{Object distance}}$$

Magnification may also be determined by comparing image size to object size. Images twice as large have a magnification of 2, whereas images half as large have a magnification of 0.5.

$$\text{Magnification} = \frac{\text{Image size}}{\text{Object size}}$$

Example 6

What is the magnification of the image produced by a +5.5 D lens if an object is placed 2 m from the lens?

$$\begin{aligned}
\text{Object distance } (u) &= 2 \text{ m} \\
\text{Object vergence } (U) &= \tfrac{1}{2} \\
U &= 0.5 \text{ D} \\
\text{Power of lens } (P) &= +5.5 \text{ D}
\end{aligned}$$

First, the image vergence and image distance must be calculated using the Vergence Equation (see below). Remember to assign a minus sign to U in all calculations for single lenses.

$$\begin{aligned}
\text{Vergence Equation:} \quad V &= U + P \\
\text{Image vergence } (V) &= (-0.5) + (+5.5) \\
V &= -0.5 + 5.5 \\
V &= +5 \text{ D} \\
\text{Image distance } (\tfrac{1}{V}) &= \tfrac{1}{5} \\
\tfrac{1}{V} &= 0.2 \text{ m}
\end{aligned}$$

$$\text{Magnification } (\frac{\text{Image distance}}{\text{Object distance}}):$$

$$= \frac{0.2}{2}$$

$$= \frac{2}{20}$$

$$= \frac{1}{10}$$

$$= 0.1$$

The image will be one-tenth the size of the object.

Example 7

What is the magnification if a plus lens creates a 10-cm-tall image of a 5-cm-tall object?

$$\text{Object size} = 5 \text{ cm}$$
$$\text{Image size} = 10 \text{ cm}$$
$$\text{Magnification} = \frac{\text{Image size}}{\text{Object size}}$$
$$= \frac{10}{5}$$
$$= 2$$

The image will be 2 times as tall as the object.

Prism Power

Please see Chapter 14 for additional details.

The power of a prism is measured in prism diopters [abbreviated as PD or with a superscript triangle (Δ)]. 1 PD or 1^Δ displaces an image toward the prism base by 1 cm at a distance of 1 m from the prism. Expressed mathematically:

$$P = \frac{C}{D}$$

Where:
- $P =$ prism power (PD or Δ)
- $C =$ displacement of real image toward prism base (cm)
- $D =$ distance of real image from prism (m)

Please see Chapter 14 for details of real and virtual images produced by prisms.

Example 8

What is the power of a prism that displaces an image 5 cm toward the base at a distance of 2 m?

$$P = \frac{C}{D}$$
$$C = 5 \text{ cm}$$
$$D = 2 \text{ m}$$
$$P = \frac{5}{2}$$
$$P = 2.5^\Delta$$

Example 9

How far is the real image displaced by a 10^Δ at a distance of 0.5 m?

$$P = \frac{C}{D}$$
$$P = 10^\Delta$$
$$D = 0.5 \text{ m}$$

$$C = (P)(D) \qquad \text{(Parentheses are used only for convenience.)}$$
$$C = (10)(0.5)$$
$$C = 5 \text{ cm}$$

Example 10

How far from a 4^Δ prism will an image be displaced 8 cm toward the prism base?

$$P = \frac{C}{D}$$
$$P = 4^\Delta$$
$$C = 8 \text{ cm}$$

To determine D, switch its position with P.

$$D = \frac{C}{P}$$
$$D = \frac{8}{4}$$
$$D = 2 \text{ m}$$

Power of Mirrors

Please see Chapter 15 for additional details.

Reflecting power of concave and convex mirrors is expressed in D, which may be related to the focal length (f) and radius of curvature (r) of the mirror in m:

$$D = \frac{1}{f_{(m)}} = \frac{2}{r_{(m)}}$$

Where:

D = reflecting power of a mirror in D
$f_{(m)}$ = focal length of a mirror in m
$r_{(m)}$ = radius of curvature of a mirror in m

Example 11

What is the power of a mirror whose f is 0.5 m?

$$D = \frac{1}{f_{(m)}}$$
$$D = \frac{1}{0.5}$$
$$D = \frac{10}{5}$$
$$D = 2 \text{ D}$$

Example 12

What is f for a mirror whose power is 2 D?

$$D = \frac{1}{f_{(m)}}$$

To determine f, switch its position with D:

$$f_{(m)} = \frac{1}{D}$$
$$f_{(m)} = \frac{1}{2}$$
$$f_{(m)} = 0.5 \text{ m}$$

Example 13

What is the power of a mirror whose r is 0.5 m?

$$D = \frac{2}{r_{(m)}}$$

$$D = \frac{2}{0.5}$$

$$D = \frac{20}{5}$$

$$D = 4 \, D$$

Example 14

What is r for a mirror whose power is 2 D?

$$D = \frac{2}{r_{(m)}}$$

To determine r, switch its position with D:

$$r_{(m)} = \frac{2}{D}$$

$$r_{(m)} = \frac{2}{2}$$

$$r_{(m)} = 1 \, m$$

Conoid of Sturm and Spherical Equivalent

Please see Chapter 20 for additional details.

The spherical equivalent of cylindrical and spherocylindrical lens prescriptions is based on the Conoid of Sturm and may be calculated by algebraically adding half the cylinder power to the sphere power.

Example 15

Cylindrical lens prescriptions:

	Plus Cylinder Form	Minus Cylinder Form
Lens prescription:	PL +0.50 x 90	+0.50 −0.50 x 180
Half cylinder power:	$\frac{0.50}{2} = +0.25$	$\frac{0.50}{2} = -0.25$
Sphere power:	0	+0.50
Spherical equivalent:	(Sphere power) + (Half cylinder power)	
	(0) + (+0.25)	(+0.50) + (−0.25)
	0 + 0.25	+0.50 −0.25
	+0.25	+0.25

Example 16

Spherocylindrical lens prescriptions:

	Plus Cylinder Form	Minus Cylinder Form
Lens prescription:	+1.50 +0.50 x 85	+2.00 -0.50 x 175
Half cylinder power:	$\frac{0.50}{2} = +0.25$	$\frac{0.50}{2} = -0.25$
Sphere power:	+1.50	+2.00

Spherical equivalent:

$$\text{(Sphere power)} + \text{(Half cylinder power)}$$

$(+1.50) + (+0.25)$	$(+2.00) + (-0.25)$
$+1.50 + 0.25$	$+2.00 - 0.25$
$+1.75$	$+1.75$

Refracting Power of a Curved Surface

Please see Chapter 22 for additional details.

The radius of curvature (r) of the cornea, and, therefore, tear film, adds the final variable to light refraction. Similarly, the power of lenses varies depending on their r.

The refracting power of a curved surface is expressed mathematically by:

$$P_{(D)} = \frac{(n_2 - n_1)}{r_{(m)}}$$

Where:

$P =$ refractive power in D
$n_1 =$ refractive index (RI) of the medium from which light is coming (first medium)
$n_2 =$ RI of the medium into which light is going (second medium)
$r =$ radius of curvature (in m) of refractive surface

Example 17

What is the power of a cornea whose r is 8.7 mm, assuming there is no tear film? (NOTE: RI of air = 1.000; RI of the cornea = 1.376; and 1 m = 1000 mm.)

$$r = 8.7 \text{ mm}$$

$$r = \frac{8.7}{1000}$$

$$r = 0.0087 \text{ m}$$

$$P_{(D)} = \frac{(n_2 - n_1)}{r_{(m)}}$$

$$P_{(D)} = \frac{(1.376 - 1.000)}{0.0087}$$

$$P_{(D)} = \frac{0.376}{0.0087}$$

$$P_{(D)} = 43.2 \text{ D}$$

Note: This is the relationship on which keratometry is based. The value of n_2 of an ophthalmometer (Keratometer, Bausch & Lomb, Rochester, NY) is standardized to 1.3375. See Chapter 22 for details.

Base Curve of Spectacle Lenses

Please see Chapter 26 for additional details.

The refracting power of a curved surface, described above, may also be applied to spectacle lenses. The anterior curved surface of spectacle lenses is termed the *base curve*, and its refracting power is determined similar to the refractive power of a curved surface:

$$P_{(D)} = \frac{(n_2 - n_1)}{r_{(m)}}$$

Where:

P =   refractive power in D
n_1 =   RI of the medium from which light is coming (air)
n_2 =   RI of the medium into which light is going (spectacle lens)
r =   base curve; radius of curvature (in m) of the anterior surface of a spectacle lens

Due to various optical relationships, described in Chapters 22 and 26, the base curve of spectacle lenses always provides plus power.

Manufacturers have standardized n_2 to 1.530, and the same formula now becomes (NOTE: the value of r is now in mm):

$$P_{(D)} = \frac{530}{r_{(mm)}}$$

Example 18

What is the power of a spectacle lens base curve whose r is 53 mm?

$$P_{(D)} = \frac{530}{r_{(mm)}}$$
$$P_{(D)} = \frac{530}{53}$$
$$P_{(D)} = +10\ D$$

Example 19

What is r for a spectacle lens base curve whose power is +6.5 D?

$$P_{(D)} = \frac{530}{r_{(mm)}}$$

Rearrange equation:

$$r_{(mm)} = \frac{530}{P_{(D)}}$$
$$r_{(mm)} = \frac{530}{6.5}$$
$$r_{(mm)} = 81.5\ mm$$

Base Curve of Contact Lenses

Please see Chapter 27 for additional details.

The refracting power of a curved surface, described above, may also be applied to contact lenses. The posterior curved surface of contact lenses is termed the base curve, and its refracting power is determined similar to the refractive power of a curved surface:

$$P_{(D)} = \frac{(n_2 - n_1)}{r_{(mm)}}$$

Where:

P =   refractive power in diopters (D)
n_1 =   RI of the medium from which light is coming (tear film)
n_2 =   RI of the medium into which light is going (contact lens)
r =   base curve; radius of curvature (in m) of the posterior surface of a contact lens

Manufacturers have standardized n_2 to 1.3375, and the same formula now becomes (NOTE: the value of r is now in mm):

$$P_{(D)} = \frac{337.5}{r_{(mm)}}$$

Example 20

What is the power of a contact lens base curve whose r is 8.4 mm?

$$P_{(D)} = \frac{337.5}{r_{(mm)}}$$

$$P_{(D)} = \frac{337.5}{8.4}$$

$$P_{(D)} = 40.17 \text{ D}$$

Example 21

What is the r of a contact lens base curve whose power is 45 D?

$$P_{(D)} = \frac{337.5}{r_{(mm)}}$$

Rearrange equation:

$$r_{(mm)} = \frac{337.5}{P_{(D)}}$$

$$r_{(mm)} = \frac{337.5}{45}$$

$$r_{(mm)} = 7.5 \text{ mm}$$

Amplitude of Accommodation

Please see Chapter 23 for additional details.

The amplitude of accommodation (ie, the amount of accommodation based on age) may be determined using the following formulae:

$$\text{Age 8 to 39:} \quad \text{amplitude} = 14 - \left(\frac{age - 8}{4}\right)$$

$$\text{Age 40 to 48:} \quad \text{amplitude} = 6 - \left\{1.5 \left(\frac{age - 40}{4}\right)\right\}$$

$$\text{Age >48:} \quad \text{amplitude} = 3 - \left\{0.5 \left(\frac{age - 48}{4}\right)\right\}$$

Example 22

What is the amplitude of accommodation of a 32-year-old?

$$\text{Age 8 to 39:} \quad \text{amplitude} = 14 - \left(\frac{age - 8}{4}\right)$$

$$\text{amplitude} = 14 - \left(\frac{32 - 8}{4}\right)$$

$$= 14 - \left(\frac{24}{4}\right)$$

$$= 14 - 6$$

$$= 8 \text{ D}$$

Example 23

What is the amplitude of accommodation of a 44-year-old?

$$\text{Age 40 to 48: } \quad \text{amplitude} = 6 - \{1.5\,(\tfrac{age - 40}{4})\}$$
$$\text{amplitude} = 6 - \{1.5\,(\tfrac{44 - 40}{4})\}$$
$$= 6 - \{1.5\,(\tfrac{4}{4})\}$$
$$= 6 - \{1.5\,(1)\}$$
$$= 6 - 1.5$$
$$= 4.5 \text{ D}$$

Example 24

What is the amplitude of accommodation of a 68-year-old?

$$\text{Age > 48: } \quad \text{amplitude} = 3 - \{0.5\,(\tfrac{age - 48}{4})\}$$
$$\text{amplitude} = 3 - \{0.5\,(\tfrac{68 - 48}{4})\}$$
$$= 3 - \{0.5\,(\tfrac{20}{4})\}$$
$$= 3 - \{0.5\,(5)\}$$
$$= 3 - 2.5$$
$$= 0.5 \text{ D}$$

Prentice's Rule, Decentration, and Induced Prism

Please see Chapters 14 and 25 for additional details.

Prentice's rule relates the amount of induced prism (in PD or $^\Delta$) to the power (in D) of the spectacle lens and the decentration (in cm) of the optical center (OC) from the pupil center.

$$\text{Induced prism}_{(\Delta \text{ or PD})} = \text{Lens power}_{(D)} \times \text{OC displacement}_{(cm)}$$

Example 25

What is the induced prism if the OC of a +10 D spectacle lens is decentered by 5 mm?

$$\text{Induced Prism}_{(\Delta \text{ or PD})} = \text{Lens Power}_{(D)} \times \text{OC Displacement}_{(cm)}$$
$$= 10 \times 0.5$$
$$= 5^\Delta$$

Example 26

How much will the OC of a +6 D spectacle lens be decentered to produce 3^Δ of induced prism?

$$\text{Induced Prism}_{(\Delta \text{ or PD})} = \text{Lens Power}_{(D)} \times \text{OC Displacement}_{(cm)}$$

Rearrange the equation:

$$\text{OC Displacement}_{(cm)} = \frac{\text{Induced Prism}_{(\Delta \text{ or PD})}}{\text{Lens Power}_{(D)}}$$
$$= \frac{3}{6}$$
$$= \frac{1}{3}$$
$$= 0.3 \text{ cm}$$

Example 27

What is the power of a spectacle lens that produces 1^Δ of induced prism when the OC is decentered by 2 mm?

$$\text{Induced Prism}_{(\Delta \text{ or PD})} = \text{Lens Power}_{(D)} \times \text{OC Displacement}_{(cm)}$$

Rearrange the equation:

$$\text{Lens Power}_{(D)} = \frac{\text{Induced Prism}_{(\Delta \text{ or PD})}}{\text{OC Displacement}_{(cm)}}$$

$$= \frac{1}{0.2}$$

$$= \frac{10}{2}$$

$$= 5\,D$$

Note: The examples shown above do not include the direction of the induced prism base because doing that requires a discussion of the prismatic effects of lenses. Please see Chapters 14 and 25 for those details.

Review Questions

1. What is the RI of a transparent medium in which light travels at a speed of 0.5×10^{10} cm/sec?

    a.   6
    b.   5
    c.   4
    d.   3

2. What is the speed of light in a transparent medium of RI of 5?

    a. 0.3×10^{10} cm/sec
    b. 6×10^{10} cm/sec
    c. 3×10^{10} cm/sec
    d. 0.6×10^{10} cm/sec

3. What is f for a lens whose power is 3.75 D?

    a.   0.27 m
    b.   2.7 m
    c.   27 m
    d.   270 m

4. What is the image vergence of an object held 2 m in front of a +5.5 D lens?

    a.   +3 D
    b.   +4 D
    c.   +5 D
    d.   +6 D

5. What is the magnification if a plus lens creates a 3-cm-tall image of a 6-cm-tall object?

    a. 0.3
    b. 5
    c. 3
    d. 0.5

6. How far is the image displaced toward the base by a 7^Δ prism at a distance of 3 m?

    a. 2.1 cm
    b. 21 cm
    c. 0.21 cm
    d. 210 cm

7. How far from a 24^Δ prism will an image be displaced 12 cm toward the prism base?

    a. 24 m
    b. 0.5 m
    c. 12 m
    d. 5 m

8. What is the power of a mirror whose r is 5 m?

    a. 0.4 D
    b. 5 D
    c. 4 D
    d. 0.5 D

9. What is the spherical equivalent of the lens prescription PL −1.00 x 165?

    a. +0.5 D
    b. −1 D
    c. +1 D
    d. −0.5 D

10. What is the power of a curved surface whose r is 7.8 mm? (Assume n_1 is 1.000 and n_2 is 1.376.)

    a. 78 D
    b. 48.2 D
    c. 7.8 D
    d. 4.82 D

11. What is r for a spectacle lens base curve whose power is +10 D?

    a. 100 mm
    b. 50 mm
    c. 53 mm
    d. 35 mm

12. What is the power of a contact lens base curve whose r is 7.8 mm? (Round off to the closest quarter D.)

    a. 48.25 D
    b. 78.25 D
    c. 43.25 D
    d. 73.25 D

13. What is the amplitude of accommodation of a 64-year-old?
      a.   0.5 D
      b.   1 D
      c.   1.5 D
      d.   2 D

14. What is the induced prism if the OC of a +5 D spectacle lens is decentered by 10 mm?
      a. 5^Δ
      b. 4^Δ
      c. 2^Δ
      d. 1^Δ

15. How much will the OC of a +0.50 D spectacle lens be decentered to produce 0.25^Δ of induced prism?
      a.   0.25 cm
      b.   0.5 cm
      c.   1 cm
      d.   1.5 cm

3

Light, Lasers, Polarization, Interference, and Fluorescence

Learning Objectives

Upon completion of this chapter, the reader should be able to:

o describe the visible portion of the electromagnetic spectrum.
o describe light as a wave and as a particle.
o describe coherence, polarization, interference, and fluorescence.

Key Points

o Light can be described as a wave and as a particle.
o Light as a wave: $c = \lambda f$.
o Light as a particle: photons.
o LASER (typically noted as "Laser"): Light Amplification by Stimulated Emission of Radiation.
o Polarization: light vibrates only in one direction.
o Light waves can interfere with each other: constructive and destructive.
o The wavelength of fluorescing light is longer than that of excitation light.
o Fluorescein sodium is an example of fluorescence. Blue excitation light has a shorter wavelength than green fluorescing light.

LIGHT

Light is the portion of the *electromagnetic spectrum* that is visible to a normal human eye.

But, what *is* light? Can you describe it to someone who has been unsighted since birth? These questions cannot be easily answered.

Instead, we take an indirect approach and describe various light phenomena by treating light both as a *wave* and as a *particle*.[1] In ophthalmology, some light phenomena are best described when light is considered to be a wave (eg, *interference*, used in *wavefront* scans for *refractive surgery*), whereas other phenomena are best described when light is considered to be a particle (eg, *fluorescence*, when *fluorescein sodium* dye is used).

Light as a Wave

Light waves are just like *ripples* and consist of *crests* and *troughs*. Such waves move at 90 degrees to the movement of the crests and troughs. As the wave moves forward, the crests and troughs move up and down—a characteristic found in surfboarding.

Light waves have many useful characteristics, some of which are important in ophthalmology.

All waves have *amplitude*, *speed* (c), *wavelength* (λ), and *frequency* (f) (Figure 3-1).

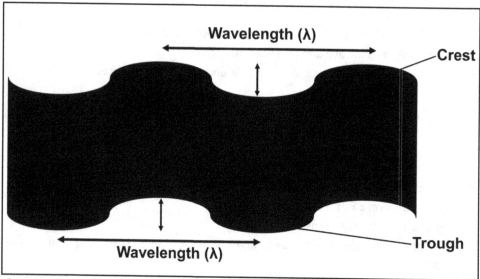

Figure 3-1. Wave shown traveling toward the right or the left. Wavelength (λ) is the distance between crests or troughs; amplitude is the height of the crest or depth of the trough (vertical arrows).

In any light wave, c, λ, and f have a specific relationship:

$$c = \lambda f$$

The *speed of light* is one of the most important constants in ophthalmology and is stated as 3×10^{10} cm/sec. If meters are used, then the speed is stated as 3×10^8 m/sec (NOTE: 1 m = 100 cm).

Note that in the equation above, the wavelength and frequency are on the same side of the equation. Therefore, these two properties of a light wave are inversely related—when one increases, the other decreases.

In ophthalmology, for example, light is the portion of the electromagnetic spectrum whose wavelength varies from approximately 400 to 700 *nanometers* (nm) and is visible to a normally functioning human eye (1 nm = 10^{-9} m = 10^{-7} cm = 10^{-6} mm).

Violet	Indigo	Blue	Green	Yellow	Orange	Red
400 nm						700 nm

Colors of this spectrum vary from the shortest wavelength (violet and blue) to the longest wavelength (red). Because of the inverse relationship of wavelength and frequency, violet and blue light have a greater frequency compared to red light, which has a lesser frequency.

For this reason, frequencies greater than violet are termed *ultraviolet* (UV) frequencies, whereas frequencies lesser than red are termed *infrared* (IR) frequencies. Wavelengths of UV waves are shorter than violet, and wavelengths of IR waves are longer than red.

Light as a Particle

Many phenomena of light may be described by treating light as a particle. Chief among these phenomena is the use of fluorescein sodium in ophthalmic tests and procedures.

Albert Einstein termed a light particle a *photon*. These particles have characteristic levels of energy and can absorb additional energy, thus entering an excited state. Excited photons release energy in the form of light of a specific wavelength, then return to resting states.

Fluorescence, in which we consider light as a particle, is described below.

LASER

Ophthalmology is a branch of medicine in which *lasers* are used very commonly. The acronym *LASER* stands for Light Amplification by Stimulated Emission of Radiation. Note that while "laser" is an acronym and should technically be written as "LASER," common usage typically notates the term as "laser," and this practice will be followed here.

Naturally radiating substances have *spontaneous emission* of radiation in which excited electrons release energy and drop to resting states. In this state, the number of excited electrons is much fewer than the number of resting electrons.

On the other hand, lasers use *stimulated emission*, which is artificially produced by exciting electrons by some method. In this state, the number of excited electrons is much greater than the number of resting electrons (termed *population inversion*).[1,2]

As excited electrons release photons and drop to resting states, the number of photons grows. Since all of the photons have the same frequency, direction of propagation, and phase, the photon beam (ie, a laser) is *monochromatic* and intense. Many different types of lasers are used in ophthalmology.[1,2]

Photocoagulation lasers are hot lasers used to thermally destroy retinal tissue in areas of leakage and/or neovascularization. The most common laser of this type is the *argon* (Ar; blue-green, 488 to 515 nm) and *krypton* (Kr; red, 647 nm). *Photodisruption* lasers are *cold lasers* used to destroy tissue by creating *microexplosions*. The neodymium:yttrium-aluminum-garnet (Nd:YAG; 1064 nm) is an example of such a laser used to open up posterior capsule opacities following cataract extraction and the implantation of a posterior chamber intraocular lens. *Photoablation* lasers use UV light to destroy some of the corneal *stroma* during refractive surgery. Such lasers, termed "*Excimer*" (excited-dimer; 193 nm), use Ar and fluorine (F) gas and are used for *PRK, LASIK, LASEK,* and *PTK.*

POLARIZATION

Natural and artificially produced light is *unpolarized* because light waves vibrate at 90 degrees in all directions to the path of light propagation. *Polarization* is achieved by using special crystals or plastic that only allow light vibrating parallel to the molecular structure to pass. Such light rays emerge vibrating in only one direction and are termed *polarized*.

Natural light reflected from various surfaces is also polarized and vibrates parallel to the surface. Vertical walls will polarize natural light vertically, whereas horizontal surfaces (eg, wet pavements and car hoods) polarize light horizontally. Typically, horizontally polarized light causes troublesome glare.

In ophthalmology, polarized light has many clinical applications. The most familiar example is the *stereo Titmus test* using the *fly, animals,* and *circles within squares*. In this familiar test, horizontally polarized glasses are used to produce images in each eye. The images are slightly displaced horizontally, and, in normal eyes, a perception of depth (stereo) is produced when the brain fuses the two images.

Polarized sunglasses are commonly prescribed, in which *vertically polarized spectacle lenses* are used to eliminate horizontally polarized light, thus decreasing glare.

Finally, a polarized *Snellen eye chart* can be used to detect malingering. In this test, the patient wears polarized glasses (eg, OD polarized at 90 degrees, and OS polarized at 180 degrees) and views the eye chart binocularly, in which alternate lines of optotypes are also polarized at 90 degrees and 180 degrees. If a patient claiming loss of vision reads all the lines, then good visual acuity is established for both eyes.

INTERFERENCE

When two waves travel together, they will interfere with each other in various ways. If the waves are exactly *in phase* (where their crests and troughs travel together), they will add to each other, and the total effect of interference will be additive. Such interference is termed *constructive* (Figure 3-2).

On the other hand, when two waves are *out of phase*, or, their crests and troughs do not travel together, they will subtract from each other, and the total effect of interference will be subtractive. Such interference is termed *destructive* (Figure 3-3).

FLUORESCENCE

As described above, Albert Einstein termed a light particle a *photon*. These particles have characteristic levels of energy and can absorb additional energy, thus entering an excited state. Excited photons release energy in the form of light of a specific wavelength, then return to resting states.

Einstein described the relationship between the wavelengths (λ) of *excitation light* (photons) and *fluorescing light* (photons) as follows:

λ of fluorescing light is longer than the λ of excitation light.

This concept is routinely applied to ophthalmic tests and procedures. The most common is the use of fluorescein sodium ophthalmic dye.

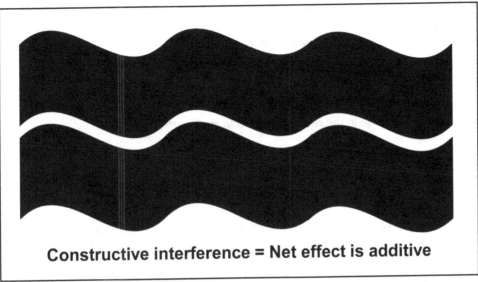

Constructive interference = Net effect is additive

Figure 3-2. Interference of waves. In constructive interference, crests and troughs of waves are in phase and match, and the net effect is additive.

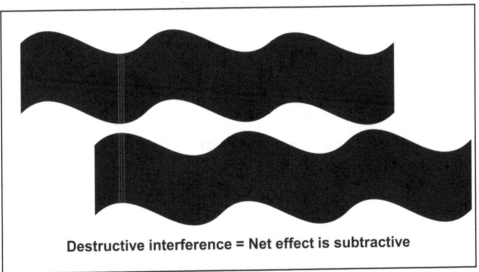

Destructive interference = Net effect is subtractive

Figure 3-3. Interference of waves. In destructive interference, crests and troughs of waves are out of phase and do not match, and the net effect is subtractive.

Remember the sequence of colors in visible light?

Violet	Indigo	Blue	Green	Yellow	Orange	Red
400 nm						700 nm

In ophthalmic practice, blue light is used to excite the orange fluorescein sodium, which then emits green light. In accordance with Einstein's theory, the λ of green light is longer than the λ of blue light.

Using the green light emitted by fluorescein is standard practice in many ophthalmic clinical procedures such as:

- obtaining *intraocular pressure* (fluorescein mires).
- assessing fit of rigid gas-permeable (RGP) contact lenses (fluorescein spread).
- assessing tear film (fluorescein break up).
- assessing breaks in the *corneal epithelium* (fluorescein staining).
- evaluating leakage in the retina (*fluorescein angiogram*).

References

1. Thall EH, Miller KM, Rosenthal P, Schechter RJ, Steinert RF, Beardsley TL. *Basic and Clinical Science Course, Section 3: Optics, Refraction, and Contact Lenses.* San Francisco, CA: American Academy of Ophthalmology; 2000.
2. Cassin B. *Fundamentals for Ophthalmic Technical Personnel.* Philadelphia, PA: WB Saunders Company; 1995.

Review Questions

1. Amplitude is a characteristic of:
   a. particles
   b. waves
   c. fluorescence
   d. polarization

2. The relationship of speed (*c*), wavelength (λ), and frequency (*f*) in a light wave may be rewritten as:
   a. $\lambda = \frac{f}{c}$
   b. $f = \frac{\lambda}{c}$
   c. $f = \lambda c$
   d. $\lambda = \frac{c}{f}$

3. Colors in the visible spectrum range in wavelength from:
   a. 300 to 600 nm
   b. 400 to 700 nm
   c. 3×10^{10} cm/sec
   d. 400 to 700 cm

4. Laser light is:
   a. coherent and monochromatic
   b. monochromatic and out of phase
   c. coherent and diffuse
   d. produced by spontaneous emission

5.   Most of the uncomfortable glare is produced by light that vibrates at:
    a.   90 degrees
    b.   45 degrees
    c.   180 degrees
    d.   135 degrees

6.   If two waves do not travel together, they will produce:
    a.   destructive interference
    b.   polarization
    c.   emission
    d.   constructive interference

7.   Fluorescence means that the:
    a.   excitation and fluorescing lights will have the same wavelengths
    b.   fluorescing light will have a longer wavelength
    c.   fluorescing and excitation lights will have the same color
    d.   excitation light will have a longer wavelength

4

SPEED OF LIGHT AND REFRACTIVE INDEX

LEARNING Objectives

Upon completion of this chapter, the reader should be able to:

o describe physical constant of speed of light.

o describe refractive index (RI).

o calculate the speed of light in various ocular tissues.

o calculate the speed of light in a medium based on its RI.

o calculate RI of a medium based on the speed of light in it.

Key Points

o The speed of light in a vacuum is a constant 3×10^{10} cm/sec.

o RI is a ratio.

o The RI of a transparent material will always be greater than 1.

SPEED OF LIGHT

The speed of light in a vacuum, such as light traveling in space from the sun to the earth, is one of the most important constants in ophthalmology.

$$3 \times 10^{10} \text{ cm/sec}$$

Since there are 100 cm in a m, the speed of light can also be expressed in m by dividing the quantity shown above by 100:

$$3 \times 10^{8} \text{ m/sec}$$

Many optical and ophthalmic calculations are based on these values. Having a good understanding of the speed of light is essential to understanding the concepts introduced below.

REFRACTIVE INDEX

Many technical staff know about spectacle lens materials such as CR-39, glass, polycarbonate, and high index. What differentiates all of these? It is *refractive index* (RI), which is different in each of these materials. The "index" in "high index" refers to the RI of the material.

RI (frequently stated as *n*) is a ratio[1]:

$$RI\ (n) = \frac{\text{Speed of light in a vacuum}}{\text{Speed of light in a medium}}$$

Note: Some references state "air" instead of "vacuum," but technically it should be "vacuum."

Since the speed of light in a vacuum is a constant, RI can be rewritten as:

$$RI\ (n) = \frac{3 \times 10^{10} \text{ cm per sec}}{\text{Speed of light in a medium}}$$

When light leaves a vacuum and meets a transparent medium such as air, tears, cornea, aqueous, lens, or vitreous, it slows down because these media are dense compared to a vacuum. The denser the medium, the more light will be slowed down. For example:

Less Dense			*More Dense*
Air	Tears, Aqueous, Vitreous	Cornea	Lens
Faster Light Travel			*Slower Light Travel*

The RI of various ocular media are listed below[1]:

Air:	1.000
Tears:	1.336
Cornea:	1.376
Crystalline lens (average):	1.386

The RI of various spectacle lenses are listed below:

Glass:	Crown:	1.523
	Flint:	1.620
	Lantal:	1.900
Plastic:	High index:	1.500 to 1.670

CALCULATIONS USING SPEED OF LIGHT AND REFRACTIVE INDEX

Since the RI is: $RI\ (n) = \dfrac{3 \times 10^{10} \text{ cm per sec}}{\text{Speed of light in a medium}}$

the speed of light can be calculated in each of the ocular tissues listed above. And, conversely, if we know the speed of light, the RI can be calculated.

$$\text{Speed of light in a medium} = \frac{3 \times 10^{10} \text{ cm per sec}}{RI\ (n)}$$

Example 1

What is the speed of light in a normal tear film? Note that the RI of tears is 1.336.

$$\text{Speed of light in a medium} = \frac{3 \times 10^{10} \text{ cm per sec}}{\text{RI } (n)}$$

$$\text{Speed of light in tears} = \frac{3 \times 10^{10} \text{ cm per sec}}{1.336}$$

$$\text{Speed of light in tears} = \frac{3}{1.336} \times 10^{10} \text{ cm/sec}$$

$$\text{Speed of light in tears} = 2.24 \times 10^{10} \text{ cm/sec}$$

Thus, light slows down approximately 25.12% in the tear film as compared to a vacuum!
Since the RI of aqueous and vitreous are the same as tears, the speed of light and the percentage at which it slows down in aqueous and vitreous is the same as it is in tears.

Example 2

What is the speed of light in a normal cornea? Note that the RI of the cornea is 1.376.

$$\text{Speed of light in a medium} = \frac{3 \times 10^{10} \text{ cm per sec}}{\text{RI } (n)}$$

$$\text{Speed of light in a normal cornea} = \frac{3 \times 10^{10} \text{ cm per sec}}{1.376}$$

$$\text{Speed of light in a normal cornea} = \frac{3}{1.376} \times 10^{10} \text{ cm/sec}$$

$$\text{Speed of light in a normal cornea} = 2.18 \times 10^{10} \text{ cm/sec}$$

Thus, light slows down approximately 27.3% in the cornea as compared to a vacuum!

Example 3

What is the speed of light in a normal crystalline lens? Note that the average RI of the crystalline lens is 1.386.

$$\text{Speed of light in a medium} = \frac{3 \times 10^{10} \text{ cm per sec}}{\text{RI } (n)}$$

$$\text{Speed of light in a normal lens} = \frac{3 \times 10^{10} \text{ cm per sec}}{1.386}$$

$$\text{Speed of light in a normal lens} = \frac{3}{1.386} \times 10^{10} \text{ cm/sec}$$

$$\text{Speed of light in a normal lens} = 2.16 \times 10^{10} \text{ cm/sec}$$

Thus, light slows down approximately 27.8% in the crystalline lens as compared to a vacuum!

With the calculations made above, we can add to the data presented previously:

Less Dense			More Dense
Air	Tears, Aqueous, Vitreous	Cornea	Lens
	2.24×10^{10} cm/sec	2.18×10^{10} cm/sec	2.16×10^{10} cm/sec
Faster Light Travel			*Slower Light Travel*

Example 4

What is the RI of a transparent substance in which light travels at a speed of 1.5 x 10^{10} cm/sec?

$$RI\ (n)\ =\ \frac{3 \times 10^{10}\ \text{cm per sec}}{\text{Speed of light in a medium}}$$

$$RI\ (n)\ =\ \frac{3 \times 10^{10}\ \text{cm per sec}}{1.5 \times 10^{10}\ \text{cm per sec}}$$

$$RI\ (n)\ =\ \frac{3}{1.5} \times \frac{10^{10}\ \text{cm per sec}}{10^{10}\ \text{cm per sec}}$$

$$RI\ (n)\ =\ \frac{3}{1.5} \times 1$$

$$RI\ (n)\ =\ 2.0$$

Example 5

Provide a mathematical explanation for the following question:

Can the RI of any medium be less than 1.0?

$$RI\ (n)\ =\ \frac{3 \times 10^{10}\ \text{cm per sec}}{\text{Speed of light in a medium}}$$

And, because the speed of light in any medium is always slower than in a vacuum, the numerator in the fraction will always be greater than the denominator:

$$RI\ (n)\ =\ \frac{3 \times 10^{10}\ \text{cm per sec}}{\text{Speed of light in a medium}}\ =\ \frac{\text{Greater}}{\text{Less}}$$

Thus, the RI of a transparent material will always be greater than 1.0.

Reference

1. Thall EH, Miller KM, Rosenthal P, Schechter RJ, Steinert RF, Beardsley TL. *Basic and Clinical Science Course, Section 3: Optics, Refraction, and Contact Lenses*. San Francisco, CA: American Academy of Ophthalmology; 2000.

Review Questions

1. The speed of light in a vacuum is:
   a. 3 x 10^{10} m/sec
   b. 3 x 10^{8} m/sec
   c. 3 x 10^{10} mm/sec
   d. 3 x 10^{8} cm/sec

2. Compared to a medium of RI 2.0, the speed of light in a medium of RI 2.5 will be:
   a. faster
   b. the same
   c. variable
   d. slower

3.   What is the speed of light in a medium of RI 3.0?
        a. 1×10^{10} cm/sec
        b. 3×10^{8} m/sec
        c. 1×10^{8} cm/sec
        d. 3×10^{10} m/sec

4.   What is the RI of a medium if the speed of light in it is 1.5×10^{8} m/sec?
        a.   1
        b.   2
        c.   3
        d.   4

5.   What is the RI of a medium if light slows down in it by 50%?
        a.   2
        b.   3
        c.   4
        d.   5

5

Snell's Law

Learning Objectives

Upon completion of this chapter, the reader should be able to:

o describe whether light bends toward or away from the normal.

o describe when light does not bend.

o describe clinical examples.

Key Points

o Snell's law: $n_{1 \text{ (or } i)} \sin i = n_{2 \text{ (or } r)} \sin r$.

o Light incident at an angle and passing from a lesser refractive index (RI) medium into a greater RI medium bends toward the normal.

o Light incident at an angle and passing from a greater RI medium into a lesser RI medium bends away from the normal.

o Light incident at 90 degrees on an interface does not bend while passing in either direction.

o Snell's law: The eye provides convergent power to light rays entering or exiting the eye.

o Snell's law: In the presence of a refractive error, a pinhole can improve visual acuity because the central rays are incident at 90 degrees and are not refracted.

Snell's Law

We have all seen these light phenomena:

o   Put water in a pan and drop a coin. As you look at the coin at an angle, the coin appears to be closer to the surface of the water than it actually is. Why does this happen?

o   As you stand at the edge of a swimming pool and look at the floor of the pool at an angle, the floor appears closer. Why does this happen?

Because light travels at different speeds in different transparent media (eg, air, water, tears, cornea, aqueous, lens, and vitreous), it bends at *interfaces* between such transparent media. Thus, light alters its path across an interface.

Snell's law describes how this bending happens, and it is the basis of all ophthalmic equipment and numerous ophthalmic tests, measurements, and protocols. A thorough understanding of Snell's law is essential for success in ophthalmology.

First, the terminology (Figure 5-1):

o   *Angle of incidence (i)* is the angle between an incident light ray and an imaginary line (called the "normal") that is drawn at 90 degrees to a transparent surface upon which light rays strike.

o   *Angle of refraction (r)* is the angle between a refracted light ray and an imaginary line (called the "normal") that is drawn at 90 degrees to a transparent surface upon which light rays strike.

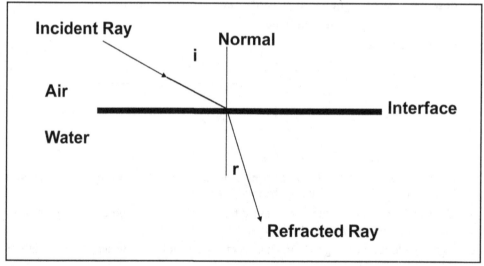

Figure 5-1. Terminology for the path of light as it passes through an interface between two transparent media of different refractive indices, such as air and water. The "normal" is an imaginary line at 90 degrees to the interface. The angle between the normal and the incident ray is the angle of incidence (*i*), whereas the angle between the normal and the refracted ray is the angle of refraction (*r*).

Snell's law states:

$$n_{1 \text{ (or } i)} \sin i = n_{2 \text{ (or } r)} \sin r$$

Where:

$n_{1 (or\ i)}$ = the RI of the medium in which light is incident
$n_{2 (or\ r)}$ = the RI of the medium in which light is refracted

Sine (abbreviated as "Sin" and pronounced "sign") is a trigonometry function present in scientific calculators.

Snell's law predicts three possibilities as light travels through an interface between two transparent media with different RI (Figure 5-2):

1. When will the refracted ray bend *toward the normal?*

2. When will the refracted ray bend *away from the normal?*

3. When will the refracted ray not bend?

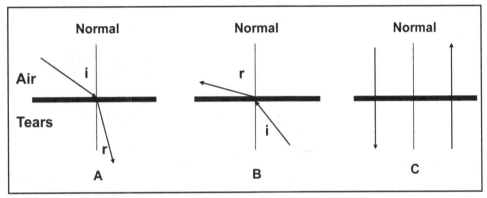

Figure 5-2. Path of light as it passes through an interface between two transparent media of different refractive indices. Light bends toward the normal when passing from a medium of lower refractive index (RI) such as air into one with a higher RI such as tears (A); it bends away from the normal when passing in the opposite direction (B), and travels unrefracted when incident at 90 degrees to the interface (C).

When Snell's law is applied to light rays passing through, say, the air, tears, cornea, and aqueous, the *refraction* of light occurs exactly as described earlier (see Figure 5-2).

First, let us recall the RI of the involved refractive media:

Air: 1.000
Tears: 1.336
Cornea: 1.376

o   The light ray traveling along the *visual axis* (termed the *central* or *chief ray*) enters the eye without being refracted since it is *incident* at 90 degrees to the interface. This effect is clinically utilized in obtaining *pinhole visual acuity.*

o   Light rays traveling parallel to the central ray go through the air-tear, tear-anterior cornea, and posterior cornea-aqueous interfaces before reaching the crystalline lens.

o   Light is refracted toward the normal at the air-tear and tear-anterior cornea interfaces. This results in *convergence.*

o   Light is refracted away from the normal at the posterior cornea-aqueous interface. This results in *divergence.*

o   Despite the divergence of light rays at the posterior cornea-aqueous interface, there is a progressive convergence of light rays as they travel through the air-tear-cornea-aqueous interfaces.

○ Since the lens and vitreous also provide convergence, the eye can be considered as a plus lens, and all characteristics of a plus lens will apply to the eye (see ahead).

Let's see how Snell's law affects light passing through the air-tear-cornea-aqueous interfaces (Figure 5-3).

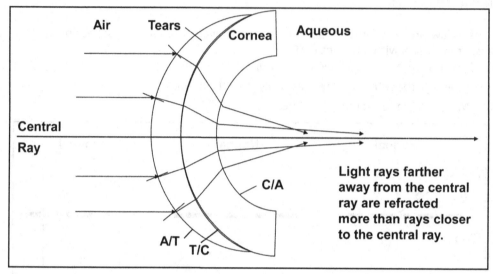

Figure 5-3. Path of light rays as they travel from air and through the tear film, the cornea, and then into the aqueous. The central (chief) ray travels along the visual axis and is not refracted since it is incident at 90 degrees. Rays parallel to the central ray are refracted toward the normal at the air-tear (A/T) and tear-cornea (T/C) interfaces, but are refracted away from the normal at the cornea-aqueous (C/A) interface.

The refraction of rays in accordance with Snell's law at the air-tear, tear-anterior cornea, and posterior cornea-aqueous interfaces may be summarized as follows:

○ The central ray is incident at 90 degrees and is not refracted at any of these interfaces.

○ At the air-tear and tear-anterior cornea interfaces, light rays bend toward the normal and provide *positive vergence* (convergence) and, therefore, *plus power.*

○ At the posterior cornea-aqueous interface, light rays bend away from the normal and provide *negative vergence* (divergence) and, therefore, *minus power.*

○ The sum total of refraction at all of these interfaces is positive vergence (convergence) and, therefore, plus power.

The two other interfaces (aqueous-anterior lens and posterior lens-vitreous) also provide positive vergence (convergence) and plus power.

Interface	Vergence	Power
Air-tear	Positive (convergence)	Plus
Tear-anterior cornea	Positive (convergence)	Plus
Posterior cornea-aqueous	Negative (divergence)	Minus
Aqueous-anterior lens	Positive (convergence)	Plus
Posterior lens-vitreous	Positive (convergence)	Plus

CLINICAL EXAMPLES

Ophthalmology has numerous examples of how Snell's law affects ocular conditions and their measurements. Some examples are explained below.

REFRACTIVE ERRORS

Light rays incident on the cornea are bent toward the normal as they travel through the air-tear, anterior cornea-aqueous, aqueous-anterior lens, and posterior lens-vitreous interfaces. All of these interfaces provide plus power. At the posterior cornea-aqueous interface, light rays are bent away from the normal, and this interface provides minus power. The net result of all of the bending (away from and toward the normal) is that all light rays eventually converge. Because of these phenomena, all of the interfaces together make the eye function like a plus lens. If the net amount of convergence is appropriate, the eye will not have a *refractive error*.

Refractive errors arise when the convergent plus power of the eye is either excessive or inadequate. Excessive plus power results in *myopia* and requires *minus lenses* to reduce the plus power of the eye, whereas inadequate plus power results in *hyperopia* and requires *plus lenses* to increase the plus power of the eye.

Astigmatism results when varying amounts of excessive or inadequate plus power are present along two axes mutually at 90 degrees to each other. This requires *cylindrical* or *spherocylindrical lenses* for correction.

INTRAOCULAR LENS CALCULATIONS

An *intraocular lens* (IOL) is implanted following removal of a natural cataractous crystalline lens. The power of the IOL must be precisely calculated in order to converge light rays on the fovea. Inadequate IOL power results in postoperative hyperopia, whereas excessive IOL power results in post operative myopia.

OVER-MINUS IN GLASSES

Refractometry should not result in excessive minus (or too little plus) power while measuring the refractive error. This caution is often stated as "do not *over-minus*," and *fogging* and *duochrome* techniques are used to ensure that this is avoided. Excessive minus power moves the image posterior to the fovea and requires that accommodation be used to move the image anteriorly and reposition it on the fovea. In *pseudophakes* and individuals with low levels of *accommodative amplitude*, this can result in blurring upon reading or fatigue. In either case, the best professional service was not provided to the patient.

REVIEW QUESTIONS

1. Refraction of light rays causes a swimming pool to appear:
    a. shallower
    b. darker
    c. deeper
    d. lighter

2.   Assuming that light rays travel at an angle into a transparent medium, all rays will:
      a.   not bend at the interface
      b.   be reflected
      c.   be stopped
      d.   bend at the interface

3.   Snell's law may be mathematically rewritten as (i = angle of incidence; r = angle of refraction):
      a. $n_2 = n_1 \frac{\sin r}{\sin i}$
      b. $n_1 = n_2 \sin i \sin r$
      c. $n_2 = n1 \sin i \sin r$
      d. $n_1 = n_2 \frac{\sin r}{\sin i}$

4.   Based on Snell's law, one factor influencing bending of light across an interface is:
      a.   RI of the two media
      b.   reflection at the interface
      c.   the normal
      d.   sunlight

5.   All light traveling at a 30-degree incident angle from a medium of lesser RI into a medium of greater RI will:
      a.   bend away from the normal
      b.   continue without refraction along the normal
      c.   bend toward the normal
      d.   be reflected

6

CRITICAL ANGLE

LEARNING Objectives

Upon completion of this chapter, the reader should be able to:

o   describe conditions for critical angle.
o   describe clinical examples.

KEY POINTS

o   Critical angle (i_c) applies when light travels from a medium of greater refractive index (RI), into a medium of lesser RI.
o   At some value of increasing angle of incidence (i), the angle of refraction (r) will have increased so much that the refracted ray grazes the interface between the two media.
o i_c is the i at which the corresponding r is maximum, and the refracted ray grazes the interface.
o   For light passing from the tears into air: i_c = 48.5 degrees.

CRITICAL ANGLE

We have all seen these, or at least heard about them!
o   In normal ocular anatomy, we cannot see the *angle structures* and must use special procedures such as *gonioscopy*.
o   *Diamonds* are more expensive and beautiful when they have greater amounts of "fire."

o   Compared to metal wire, fiber optics transmit greater amounts of data by using light. Hence, a *fiber optic cable* is the best conveyor of data for HDTVs.

How do all of these work?

Critical angle (i_c) applies only when light travels from a medium of greater refractive index (RI), such as water, cornea, or tears, into a medium of lesser RI, such as air (Figure 6-1).

o   As light travels from a medium of greater RI, such as water, cornea, or tears, and into a medium of lower RI, such as air, light bends away from the normal.

o   As the angle of incidence (*i*) increases, the angle of refraction (*r*) also increases.

o   As *i* further increases, *r* will also continue to increase.

o   As *r* continues to increase, at some value of *i* the *r* will have increased so much that the refracted ray grazes the interface between the two media.

o   At this stage, *r* will be of maximum value.

o   Therefore, the i_c is the *i* at which the corresponding *r* is maximum and the refracted ray grazes the interface.

o   In most texts, including this (see Figure 6-1 C), *r* is commonly stated as "90 degrees."

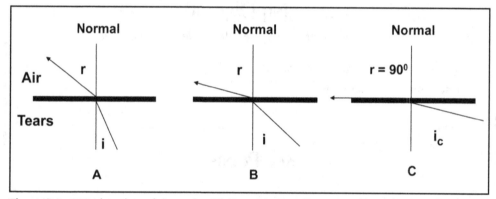

Figure 6-1. Critical angle and the path of light as it passes from a medium of greater refractive index (RI) such as tears to a medium of lower RI such as air. Light bends away from the normal (A); as the angle of incidence (*i*) increases, the angle of refraction (*r*) also increases (B). When *i* increases so that the refracted ray grazes the interface, *i* is termed the critical angle (i_c) and *r* is of maximum value, here shown as 90 degrees (C).

We can also mathematically rewrite Snell's law and derive a formula for the i_c (assume Sin 90 = 1):

Snell's law is:	$n_1 \, Sin \, i = n_2 \, Sin \, r$
Rewriting for i_c:	$n_1 \, Sin \, i_c = n_2 \, Sin \, 90$
Assuming Sin 90 = 1:	$n_1 \, Sin \, i_c = n_2 \, 1$
:	$n_1 \, Sin \, i_c = n_2$
Solving for Sin i_c:	$Sin \, i_c = \frac{n_2}{n_1}$

Thus, the formula for the i_c becomes:

$$Sin \, i_c = \frac{n_2}{n_1}$$

We can now apply this to the eye since we know the RI of the ocular media. First, let us recall the RI of the involved refractive surfaces:

Air: 1.000
Tears: 1.336

Thus, for light passing from the tears (n_1) and into the air (n_2):

$$\text{Sin } i_c = \frac{n_2}{n_1} = \frac{1.000}{1.336} = 0.7485$$

Since "Sin i_c = 0.7485," we can use a scientific calculator to find the value of "i_c," which is 48.5 degrees. This means that as long as light is incident at angles less than i_c, it will be able to emerge into air. So, what happens if the angle of incidence is increased and is greater than i_c?

Read on!

Review Questions

1. When light travels from the air and into the eye:
    a.   the i_c can be calculated
    b. $r > i$
    c.   all light will be reflected
    d. i_c will not apply

2. What is the speed of light in a medium whose RI is 3.000?
    a. 9×10^{10} m/sec
    b. 0.3×10^{10} cm/sec
    c. 1×10^{8} m/sec
    d. 0.1×10^{10} cm/sec

3. What is the value of Sin i_c if light travels from a medium of RI 2.000 into a medium of RI 1.000? (Assume Sin r = 1.0.)
    a.   1
    b.   0.5
    c.   2
    d.   0.3

4. What will happen if light travels from a medium of RI 2.000 into a medium of RI 1.000 and is incident at an angle of 30 degrees?
    a. $r < 30$ degrees
    b. $i < 30$ degrees
    c. $r > 30$ degrees
    d. $i > 30$ degrees

5. What will happen if light travels from a medium of RI 1.000 into a medium of RI 2.000 and is incident at an angle of 30 degrees?
    a. $r < 30$ degrees
    b. $i < 30$ degrees
    c. $r > 30$ degrees
    d. $i > 30$ degrees

7

TOTAL INTERNAL REFLECTION

LEARNING Objectives

Upon completion of this chapter, the reader should be able to:

o describe conditions of total internal reflection.
o describe clinical and other examples.

KEY POINTS

o Total internal reflection (TIR) requires that 1) light pass from a medium of greater refractive index (RI) into a medium of lesser RI; and 2) the angle of incidence (i) exceed the critical angle (i_c).
o In TIR, all light is reflected back into the medium of greater RI, and none is refracted into the medium of lesser RI.
o Ophthalmic examples of TIR include angle structures and keratoconus.
o An industrial example of TIR is a fiber optic cable.
o A cosmetic example of TIR is a diamond.

CRITICAL ANGLE REVIEW

In the previous chapter we learned that i_c applies only when light travels from a medium of greater RI such as water, cornea, or tears into a medium of lesser RI such as air.

An example of this condition is when light from the angle structures travels through the aqueous, cornea, and tears, and into air.

In this condition, as long as light is incident at angles less than i_c (48.5 degrees), it will emerge into air. What happens if the i is increased and is greater than i_c?

TOTAL INTERNAL REFLECTION

The conditions for i_c are also required for *total internal reflection* (TIR).

TIR can only occur when light travels from a medium of greater RI into a medium of lesser RI. At the end of the previous chapter, we asked what would happen to light if the *i* exceeded i_c.

In this condition, when $i > i_c$, ALL light is *reflected* back into the medium of greater RI, and NO light is refracted into the medium of lesser RI (Figure 7-1). This condition is termed total internal reflection.

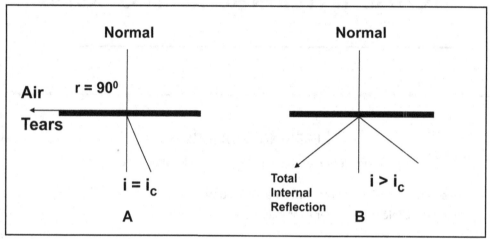

Figure 7-1. Total internal reflection. When the angle of incidence (*i*) is the critical angle (i_c), the refracted ray grazes the interface and the angle of refraction (*r*) is of maximum value, here shown to be 90 degrees (A). When *i* exceeds i_c, no refraction occurs because all light is reflected back into the first medium in total internal reflection (B).

Therefore, the following conditions must be met for light to undergo TIR:
○   Light travels from a medium of greater RI into a medium of lesser RI.
○   The *i* must exceed the i_c.

Since light from the angle structures exceeds the i_c (48.5 degrees), the conditions of TIR are fulfilled, light is reflected back into the anterior chamber, and angle structures are not visible without gonioscopy. In cases of *keratoconus* and a well-developed *inferior cone, i* is less than i_c, and the angle structures may be visible without gonioscopy.

CLINICAL AND OTHER APPLICATIONS

ANGLE STRUCTURES

In patients with anatomically normal corneas, the angle structures are not visible unless special procedures such as gonioscopy are used. Gonioscopes are large contact lenses that are manually held against the cornea by the ophthalmologist in order to view and evaluate the angle and its structures.

To view the angle structures, the conditions of TIR must be removed. The most efficient way to accomplish this is to remove air as a refractive medium. This can be done by 1) applying *hydroxylpropylmethylcellulose* (Goniosol), whose RI is similar to tears, to the cornea on a mirrored *Goldmann lens* or non-mirrored *Koeppe lens*; or 2) using tears to contact a *Zeiss-Posner lens* against the cornea. In both methods, light emerging from the angle structures does not encounter air and the *i* does not exceed the i_c. As a result, TIR does not occur and light leaves the anterior chamber, making the angle structures visible.

Fiber Optics

Fiber optic cables, which transmit greater amounts of data than conventional cables, use TIR as their process.

An optic cable actually consists of two cables—one inside the other. The inner cable has a greater RI, whereas the outer cable has a lesser RI. Thus, as light passes the interface between the two cables, the refracted ray would normally bend away from the normal. Since *i* exceeds i_c, all light is reflected back as TIR and emerges at the other end of the cable with larger amounts of data.

Diamonds

The "fire" of diamonds is well known, and the greater the fire, the more expensive the diamond.

Natural diamonds have eight faces, and the crystal does not appear lustrous in its natural state. To convert this into an expensive gemstone, dozens of faces at varying angles are cut and polished on the crystal. In this way, a non-lustrous natural crystal is transformed into a desirable gemstone.

As light travels past the interface between the diamond and air on each crystal face, the refracted ray would normally bend away from the normal. However, diamond faces are cut and polished at such an angle that *i* exceeds i_c and all light is reflected back into the diamond as TIR. As the diamond is turned, and, depending on the lighting conditions, *i* is less than i_c in some of the crystal faces, and the refracted rays emerge from those faces as brilliant light ("fire").

The more expensive diamonds have greater numbers of faces and more places on the crystal where the "fire" may be observed.

Review Questions

1. During TIR:
    a. the refracted ray bends toward the normal
    b. light goes from air into a gemstone
    c. the refracted ray bends away from the normal
    d. there is no refraction

2. If light is passing from a medium of RI 1.523 into a medium of RI 1.376 and is incident at an angle of 50 degrees, how will the light behave if the i_c is 40 degrees?
    a. refracted rays will bend away from the normal
    b. rays will be totally internally reflected
    c. refracted rays will graze the interface between the media
    d. refracted rays will bend toward the normal

3.   An example of TIR is light passing:
    a.   from the angle structures toward the outside of the eye
    b.   from air into a fiber optic cable
    c.   from air into a diamond
    d.   to the angle structures from the outside of the eye

4.   A large uncut diamond:
    a.   has dozens of crystal faces
    b.   has lots of fire
    c.   will not display TIR
    d.   may be expensive

5.   Angle structures may be visible without gonioscopy in:
    a.   against-the-rule astigmatism
    b.   a corneal cone
    c.   hypoglobus
    d.   microcornea

TYPES OF LENSES

LEARNING Objectives

Upon completion of this chapter, the reader should be able to:

o   describe characteristics and uses of plus lenses.
o   describe characteristics and uses of minus lenses.

KEY POINTS

o   A lens is a refracting device in which at least one surface is curved.

o   Light refracted by a lens will either converge or diverge.

o   Plus lenses converge light and are similar to two prisms placed base to base.

o   Minus lenses diverge light and are similar to two prisms placed apex to apex.

o   A spherical lens has the same power in all directions and corrects myopia or hyperopia.

o   Cylindrical lenses have plane and curved surfaces and correct astigmatic ametropia.

o   Astigmatism is produced due to a cylindrical effect by the cornea and/or crystalline lens.

o   Five types of astigmatism may be identified.

o   Presbyopia is the gradual loss of accommodation with increasing age.

WHAT IS A LENS?

A lens is a *refracting device* in which at least one surface is *curved*. If both refracting surfaces are curved, the lens is termed a *meniscus lens*. Common examples are spectacle, trial, and contact lenses. The *optic axis* (also, *principal axis* or *lens axis*) passes through the center of the lens. Light traveling along the optic axis is at 90 degrees to the lens surface and, according to Snell's law, travels through the air-lens interface without being refracted. Everywhere else on the lens, the angle of incidence (*i*) is not at 90 degrees, and light is refracted along the air-lens interface according to Snell's law (see Chapter 5).

Because of curved surfaces, lenses also have power. The greater the curvature, the greater the *lens power* and the refraction of light as it travels through the lens. The refracted light will either converge or diverge, and both types of refracted light are termed *vergence*. Convergence is termed positive or plus vergence and provides plus power, whereas divergence is termed negative or minus vergence and provides minus power.

PLUS LENSES

If the middle of the curved refracting surface bows away from the center of the lens, the curved refracting surface has plus power, and the lens is termed a *plus lens*. Such lenses may be considered similar to two *prisms* (see Chapter 14 for prisms) placed base to base (Figure 8-1).

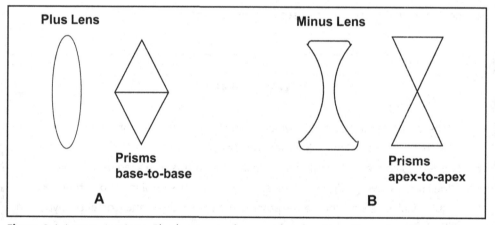

Figure 8-1. Lenses as prisms. Plus lenses may be considered as two prisms placed base to base (A); whereas minus lenses may be considered as two prisms placed apex to apex (B).

Due to their *prismatic effect* and Snell's law, plus lenses refract light toward the *optic axis*. The net result of doing so is that plus lenses converge light. Converging light is also termed *positive (plus) vergence* and produces images that are inverted and magnified. Since plus lenses provide plus power, they are used to correct hyperopia, in which plus power of the eye is inadequate and needs to be increased.

When a plus lens moves from the *spectacle plane* to the *corneal plane* (ie, when contact lenses are worn in place of spectacles), the plus lens loses plus power. This loss of plus power must be compensated when contact lenses are recommended for refractive errors of +4 D and greater. This compensation is termed *vertex correction* (see Chapter 27).

The loss of plus power is further increased when a lens moves closer to the *retinal plane* (ie, when anterior chamber or posterior chamber intraocular lenses [IOLs] are implanted). In addition, once implanted, if an IOL moves, it changes the optics, thus inducing refractive errors (see Power of Intraocular Lens Implants on page 57).

Principal characteristics of plus lenses are listed in Table 8-1.

Minus Lenses

If the middle of the curved refracting surface bows toward the center of the lens, the curved refracting surface has minus power, and the lens is termed a *minus lens*. Such lenses may be considered similar to two prisms (see Chapter 14 for prisms) placed apex to apex (see Figure 8-1).

Due to their prismatic effect and Snell's law, minus lenses refract light away from the optic axis. The net result of doing so is that minus lenses diverge light. Diverging light, also termed *negative (minus) vergence*, produces images that are upright and reduced. Since minus lenses provide minus power, they are used to correct myopia in which plus power of the eye is excessive and needs to be decreased.

When a minus lens moves from the spectacle plane to the corneal plane (ie, when contact lenses are worn in place of spectacles), the minus lens gains minus power. This gain of minus power must be compensated when contact lenses are recommended for refractive errors of −4 D and greater. This compensation is termed *vertex correction* (see Chapter 27).

Principal characteristics of minus lenses are listed in Table 8-1.

Table 8-1		
Characteristic	**Plus Lens**	**Minus Lens**
Thickness variations between center and periphery of lens	Thicker in center; thinner at periphery	Thinner in center; thicker at periphery
Image-object relationship (magnification or reduction)	Magnifies images	Reduces images
Change in power as lens is moved away from the eye	Plus power increases	Minus power decreases
Image movement as lens is moved sideways along axis 180, or up and down along axis 90	Against motion[1]	With motion[1]
Lens shape and prisms	Two prisms placed base to base	Two prisms placed apex to apex
Refractive error corrected	Hyperopia	Myopia

[1]This should not be confused with the motion of the streak observed during retinoscopy.

Spherical Lenses

Spherical (frequently abbreviated to sphere) *lenses* have spherical surfaces and bend light with the same power in all directions. In clinical practice, the term *axis* or *meridian* is used to denote the power direction.

Refracted rays steadily converge or diverge, thus creating blur circles that gradually become smaller until they come to a *point focus*, which is the location of the best focus and the sharpest image. The point focus image is also termed a *stigmatic image*. Spherical lenses are used to correct stigmatic ametropia such as hyperopia and myopia.

In clinical practice such as in glasses or contact lenses, spherical lenses are denoted by *sphere power*, and abbreviated SPH or Sph (eg, +3.00 SPH; –2.50 Sph).

CYLINDRICAL LENSES

Cylindrical (frequently abbreviated to cylinder or cyl) lenses have plane and curved surfaces and do not bend light with the same power in all directions.

The *plane surface* has no curvature and no power, and is called the *cylinder axis*. It is also the location of the image produced by a cylindrical lens. The curved surface has curvature and power, and is called the *power meridian*. Its image forms along the cylinder axis. In cylindrical lenses, the cylinder axis and power meridian are oriented at 90 degrees to each other, and the lens orientation is denoted by the cylinder axis.

The image in a cylindrical lens does not form a point focus but rather a *line focus*, and the image is termed an *astigmatic image*. Cylindrical lenses are used to correct *astigmatic ametropia*, which may be present by itself or in combination with hyperopia and myopia.

Cylindrical lenses can be plus or minus lenses and will display characteristics of those lenses similar to spherical lenses (see the sections above).

In clinical practice such as in glasses or contact lenses, cylindrical lenses are denoted by a cylinder axis and *cylinder power* (eg, +3.00 +1.00 x 90):

Sphere Power	Cylinder Power		Cylinder Axis
+3.00	+1.00	x	90

CLINICAL EXAMPLES

EMMETROPIA

The human eye may be considered as having plus power and imparting positive (plus) vergence to incident light rays. If the plus power is appropriate, the sharpest image will be located on the fovea and, assuming there are no other abnormal conditions, the visual acuity will be the best.

Such a condition is termed *emmetropia*, which means the patient does not have a refractive error and does not need corrective lenses. However, such patients might still need presbyopic correction (see ahead), which is not considered to be a refractive error, but an effect of aging.

The glasses and contact lens prescription for emmetropia is noted as:

PL Sphere
(Sphere is frequently abbreviated as SPH or Sph)

AMETROPIA

If the plus power is inappropriate, then a refractive error is present and the patient will need corrective lenses, which is the case in *ametropia* (Table 8-2).

Table 8-2			
Plus Power of Eye	**Refractive Error**	**Corrective Lens**	**Example**
Excess	Myopia	Minus (to reduce plus power)	–4.25 Sph
Inadequate	Hyperopia	Plus (to add more plus power)	+4.25 Sph

Astigmatism

Astigmatism is a refractive condition in which a line focus image is produced due to a cylindrical effect by the cornea and/or crystalline lens. Astigmatism may be present alone and corrected by a cylindrical lens, or in combination with myopia or hyperopia and corrected by spherocylindrical lenses.

Five types of astigmatism may be identified with their own characteristic corrective lenses (Table 8-3).

Table 8-3			
Astigmatism	**Plus Power**	**Corrective Lens**	**Examples of Prescriptions**
Simple Myopic (SMA)	Appropriate along one axis; excessive 90 degrees away	Minus cylindrical	PL –1.00 x 180 A similar optical effect is obtained by using a minus spherical and a plus cylindrical lens: –1.00 +1.00 x 90
Simple Hyperopic (SHA)	Appropriate along one axis; inadequate 90 degrees away	Plus cylindrical	PL +1.00 x 90 A similar optical effect is obtained by using a plus spherical and a minus cylindrical lens: +1.00 –1.00 x 180
Compound Myopic (CMA)	Excessive along both axes	Minus spherical and minus cylindrical	–2.00 –1.00 x 180 A similar optical effect is obtained by using a minus spherical and a plus cylindrical lens: –3.00 +1.00 x 90
Compound Hyperopic (CHA)	Inadequate along both axes	Plus spherical and plus cylindrical	+2.00 +1.00 x 90 A similar optical effect is obtained by using a plus spherical and a minus cylindrical lens: +3.00 –1.00 x 180
Mixed (MA)	Excessive along one axis; inadequate 90 degrees away	Minus or plus spherical and cylindrical	+1.00 –3.00 x 180 or –2.00 +3.00 x 90

Presbyopia

The gradual loss of accommodation (accommodative amplitude) with increasing age is termed *presbyopia*. Maximum accommodation of +14 D is present in a normal eye up to age 8.[1] Between ages 8 and 40, accommodation is lost at the rate of +1 D per 4 years, which equals to +6 D of accommodation remaining at age 40. Between ages 40 and 48, accommodation is lost at the rate of +1.5 D per 4 years, which equals to +3 D remaining at age 48. After age 48, accommodation is lost at the rate of +0.5 D per 4 years, resulting in zero accommodation at age 72.

So, how do we decide what *reading add* power to recommend?

Typically, a patient will hold the reading material at 33 cm, which equals a dioptric power of 3 D. Calculate the accommodation for the patient's age from the details presented above. Deduct half of the accommodation from 3 D. The remainder is the most suitable reading add power for 33 cm.

Example 1

A 56-year-old patient needs a bifocal reading add, and holds reading material at 33 cm.

$$
\begin{aligned}
\text{Reading distance} &= 33 \text{ cm} \\
&= \frac{100}{33} \\
&= +3 \text{ D}
\end{aligned}
$$

$$
\begin{aligned}
\text{Available accommodation at 56} & \\
\text{(calculate from data above)} &= +2 \text{ D} \\
\text{Use half of available accommodation} &= +1 \text{ D} \\
\text{Deduct from reading distance} &= +3 - (+1) \\
&= +3 - 1 \\
&= 2 \\
\text{Reading add} &= +2 \text{ D}
\end{aligned}
$$

At a reading distance significantly different from 33 cm, a more precise method must be followed. The more precise way is to measure the monocular accommodative amplitudes of the OD and OS, calculate the average, and deduct half of that from the *accommodative need* using a *Prince Rule*. An advanced textbook in ophthalmology should be consulted to obtain details of this procedure.

Example 2

A 56-year-old patient needs a bifocal reading add, and holds reading material at 25 cm.

$$
\begin{aligned}
\text{Reading distance} &= 25 \text{ cm} \\
&= \frac{100}{25} \\
&= +4 \text{ D} \\
\text{Accommodative amplitude OD (measured)} &= +1.25 \text{ D} \\
\text{Accommodative amplitude OS (measured)} &= +1.75 \text{ D} \\
\text{Accommodative amplitude average} &= \frac{+1.25 +1.75}{2} \\
&= \frac{+3}{2} \\
&= +1.5 \text{ D} \\
\text{Use half of available accommodation} &= +0.75 \text{ D} \\
\text{Deduct from reading distance} &= +4 - (+0.75) \\
&= +4 - 0.75 \\
&= +3.25 \\
\text{Reading add} &= +3.25 \text{ D}
\end{aligned}
$$

Thus, if a +2 D reading add power was recommended based on age but not need (as in Example 1), objects will appear blurry. Instead, the more precise method based on need results in a reading add of +3.25 D.

Power of Intraocular Lens Implants

As described above, all plus lenses lose plus power as they are moved toward the retinal plane.

This concept may be utilized in understanding the optics of an IOL implanted in the posterior chamber (PC-IOL). In patients with 1 D or less of preop refractive error, minor astigmatism, and an axial length of approximately 24 mm, the power of the required IOL might be as high as +23 D. Why is this, if the power of a normal crystalline lens is +19 D? Also, if an anterior chamber IOL (AC-IOL) is indicated, why does it require much less power?

The reasons may be deduced from the position of the IOL. A successfully implanted PC-IOL rests against the original posterior capsule. Thus, its center is slightly posterior to the original crystalline lens, and the PC-IOL is closer to the retina. It effectively has less plus power, which must be compensated by using a PC-IOL of greater plus power. On the other hand, if an AC-IOL is required, then its center will be much farther from the retina than the original crystalline lens. It effectively has more plus power, which must be compensated by using an AC-IOL of lesser plus power.

What happens to vision when a PC-IOL moves anteriorly due to capsule shrinkage? A well-positioned PC-IOL producing emmetropia forms images on the fovea. As the IOL moves anteriorly and away from the retina, it effectively has more plus power, thus moving images anteriorly into the vitreous. An eye with excess plus power is myopic, so the anterior movement of a PC-IOL induces a *myopic shift*.

Reference

1. Thall EH, Miller KM, Rosenthal P, Schechter RJ, Steinert RF, Beardsley TL. *Basic and Clinical Science Course, Section 3: Optics, Refraction, and Contact Lenses.* San Francisco, CA: American Academy of Ophthalmology; 2000.

Review Questions

1.   What characteristics do plus and minus lenses have?
     a.   plus lenses magnify images and display against motion of the image, whereas minus lenses reduce image size and display with motion of the image
     b.   plus lenses are thicker at the periphery
     c.   plus lenses reduce image size and display against motion of the image, whereas minus lenses magnify images and display with motion of the image
     d.   minus lenses are thicker in the middle

2.   All spherical lenses:
    a.   have different powers along various meridians
    b.   have the same power in all meridians
    c.   only converge light
    d.   only diverge light

3.   The image in a cylindrical lens:
    a.   forms 30 degrees to the axis
    b.   forms 45 degrees to the axis
    c.   forms a line focus
    d.   does not form

4.   An example of a prescription to correct simple myopic astigmatism is:
    a.   −2.00 +1.00 x 180
    b.   −2.00 +2.00 x 90
    c.   +2.00 −1.00 x 90
    d.   +2.00 +1.00 x 180

5.   An example of a prescription to correct mixed astigmatism is:
    a.   −2.00 +3.00 x 45
    b.   +3.00 +2.00 x 135
    c.   −2.00 −3.00 x 45
    d.   +3.00 +3.00 x 135

REFLECTION AND MIRRORS

LEARNING Objectives

Upon completion of this chapter, the reader should be able to:

o describe the Law of Reflection.
o describe the characteristics of concave and convex mirrors.
o describe clinical and other examples.

KEY POINTS

o The Law of Reflection states that the angle of incidence (i) = angle of reflection (r).
o Mirrors reverse the direction of light travel.
o Convex mirrors diverge light rays similar to minus lenses.
o Concave mirrors converge light rays similar to plus lenses.
o Plane mirrors do not diverge or converge light similar to plano lenses.

LAW OF REFLECTION

Have you ever played billiards? If so, have you noticed that the white cue ball is deflected from the table bank or from other balls at the same angle at which it impacted them? And furthermore, the greater the angle at which the ball impacts the bank or another ball, the greater the angle at which it is deflected?

Incident and reflected light behave in much the same way.

Stand in front of a mirror in your bathroom and shine a light so the beam is incident at 90 degrees to the mirror. The light will be reflected back at the same angle (90 degrees), and you will experience a lot of glare. Now, move the light to one side so that the angle of incidence (the angle between the incident light rays and an imaginary line, drawn at 90 degrees to the mirror) increases. You will notice that the reflected beam bounces off of the mirror at an angle, and that the angle of reflection (the angle between the reflected light rays and an imaginary line, drawn at 90 degrees to the mirror) increases as you continue to move the light to the side.

The *Law of Reflection* states:

o   the angle of incidence (*i*) = angle of reflection (*r*)

o   *r* is independent of the refractive index (RI) of the transparent medium

This law applies whenever light is reflected off of a surface—shiny or otherwise. Reflection and reflected light play a great role in measurements using ophthalmic instruments, many of which use *convex* or *concave mirrors*.

MIRRORS

All *mirrors* reverse the direction of light travel, and concave and convex mirrors also change the degree of convergence and divergence of light. Since light does not pass through a mirror, the concepts of RI and Snell's law do not apply to mirrors.

The principal characteristics of mirrors are shown in Table 9-1.

Table 9-1			
Mirror	**Reflected Light**	**Equivalent Lens**	**Image Produced by Mirror**
Convex	Rays diverge	Minus	Reduced and upright
Concave	Rays converge	Plus	Magnified and upright if the object is closer than the focal length of the mirror or magnified and inverted if the object is farther than the focal length of the mirror
Plane	Unchanged	Plano	Upright and same size as object

CLINICAL EXAMPLES

KERATOMETRY

The tear film on a normal cornea reflects light similar to a convex mirror. The reflected light is divergent, and the image (mires, or circles observed through the eyepiece) is reduced and upright. This concept is used in measuring corneal curvature with an *ophthalmometer* (Keratometer).

A steeper cornea has more divergent power than a flatter cornea. The light reflected from a steeper cornea produces smaller images (mires) than those produced from a flatter cornea. Since tears are necessary for proper reflection, dry eyes result in distorted mires during *keratometry*.

Computed Corneal Topography

Computed corneal topography (CCT) is based on the *Placido disc,* a large circular board with concentric black and white rings on a white background and a central opening for viewing the cornea. As light shines on the disc and the patient's cornea, the examiner views the cornea and observes images of the concentric rings produced on the cornea.

The same process is used in CCT (hence the concentric rings at the center of which the patient gazes), and may be viewed in real time in the *photokeratoscope view.* In this view, a steeper cornea shows rings spaced closer together while a flatter cornea shows rings spaced farther apart. The computer program simply does the calculations and presents the data using artificial colors in an axial view. Simulated dioptric readings may be obtained in the keratometry and numerical views.

Retinoscopy for Evaluating Hyperopia

The light from the retinoscope is termed the *intercept,* whereas the light reflected from the fundus and observed through the pupil is termed the *streak.* This terminology will be followed ahead. Standard textbooks (see References) should be consulted for additional details of *retinoscopy.*

The *plane mirror* in a *streak retinoscope* reflects light from the lamp, which can be placed closer or farther from a plus lens by moving the *retinoscope collar* vertically [downward in a Copeland (Stereo Optical Co., Inc, Chicage, IL) and upward in a Welch-Allyn (Skaneateles, NY)] while observing with motion of the streak. Moving the collar vertically produces convergent light (plus power) from the retinoscope, and thus is used to *estimate hyperopia* along each meridian separately.[1]

At some position of the collar, the streak will appear the sharpest. This is termed a *concave-mirror effect* and produces an *enhanced streak (sharply focused streak).* An enhanced streak can only be used when with motion is observed, indicating the presence of hyperopia. Myopia (against motion of the streak) already has excessive convergent (plus) power, and providing additional plus power will only increase myopia and against motion of the streak.

The maximum convergent (plus) power that can be provided by enhancing the streak in this manner is +5 D, and it requires that the retinoscope collar be moved vertically halfway in order to produce the sharpest streak. Moving the collar vertically ¼ of the way provides approximately +2.5 D. There are no markings denoting the ¼ or halfway positions of the collar, so the best approximation must be used.

Clinically, an enhanced streak is used in estimating the amount of hyperopia along one meridian. The examiner should monitor the vertical movement of the collar to obtain an estimation of the degree of hyperopia[1]:

o   moving the collar ½ way = approximately +5 D of hyperopia

o   moving the collar ¼ way = approximately +2.5 D of hyperopia

By evaluating the two meridians, the total hyperopic refractive error can be estimated, and a lens correction can be derived for the refractive error.

Although most ophthalmic medical personnel (OMP) do not routinely use the retinoscope in an enhanced-streak mode, this is a very useful skill to develop and incorporate into clinical applications.

Gonioscopy

Gonioscopy is used to observe the angle structures that are not visible through a normal cornea due to total internal reflection (TIR) (see Chapter 7). Gonioscopes are large contact lenses that are manually held against an anesthetized cornea by the ophthalmologist in order to view and evaluate the angle and its structures.

Goldmann and Zeiss-Posner gonioscopes have plane mirrors placed at various angles to the visual axis. When the contact lens is held in place, the examiner looks at the mirror and can view the angle and its structures. Since these mirrors are plane, the reflected light does not diverge or converge, but remains unchanged (see Table 9-1).

Lasers

Note that, while "laser" is an acronym and should technically be written as "LASER," common usage typically notates the term as "laser," and this practice will be followed here.

Lasers (see Chapter 3) produce a coherent, monochromatic light of one wavelength (eg, the diode lasers used as pointers during a lecture). To do this, light of one wavelength must be produced and the population of energized particles must be increased in a process termed *optical pumping*.[2]

Lasers produce optical pumping by bouncing energized particles between two concave mirrors, one of which has a small central opening. As light bounces between the two mirrors, it is concentrated, and part of that light leaves through the central opening as a laser beam.

Other Ophthalmic Instruments

Many ophthalmic instruments use mirrors of one kind or another. Table 9-2 summarizes commonly used ophthalmic instruments that use mirrors and are available in most examination lanes and clinics.

Table 9-2	
Instrument	**Type of Mirror**
Snellen eye chart projector	Concave
Snellen eye chart mirrors	Plane
Slit lamp (biomicroscope)	Plane
Worth 4-dot flashlight	Concave
Auto-refractor	Concave
Humphrey Field Analyzer	Convex for gaze tracking
Brightness Acuity Test	Bowl functions like a concave mirror
Exophthalmometer	Plane
Corneal alignment (Phoropter; Bausch & Lomb, Rochester, NY)	Plane

Non-Ophthalmic Mirrors

Many commonly used non-ophthalmic devices use mirrors (Table 9-3).

Device	Type of Mirror
Table 9-3	
Automobile and truck passenger-side mirror	Convex
Automobile and truck rear-view mirror	Plane
Automobile and truck driver-side mirror	Plane
Security (buildings and vehicles)	Convex
Security (inspecting under vehicles)	Plane
Traffic (intersections and hallways)	Convex
Flashlights	Concave
Bathroom and dressing	Plane
Shaving and makeup	Concave
Dental	Plane
Microscopes	Plane
Astronomical telescopes	Concave

References

1. Corboy JM. *The Retinoscopy Book: An Introductory Manual for Eye Care Professionals.* Thorofare, NJ: SLACK Incorporated; 2003.
2. Cassin B. *Fundamentals for Ophthalmic Technical Personnel.* Philadelphia, PA: WB Saunders Company; 1995.

Review Questions

1. Angle of incidence (i) = angle of reflection (r) is known as:
   a. Snell's law
   b. refractive index (RI)
   c. total internal reflection (TIR)
   d. Law of Reflection

2. One characteristic of all mirrors is that they:
   a. reverse the direction of light travel
   b. provide plus power
   c. provide no power
   d. provide minus power

3. Convex mirrors are similar to:
   a. plus lenses
   b. minus lenses
   c. no lenses
   d. plano lenses

4.   Concave mirrors are similar to:
    a.   plus lenses
    b.   minus lenses
    c.   no lenses
    d.   plano lenses

5.   Examples of use of mirrors include:
    a.   retinoscopy, gonioscopy, and slit lamp
    b.   keratometry, trial lenses, and retinoscopy
    c.   computed corneal topography, retinoscopy, and Ishihara
    d.   retinoscopy, gonioscopy, and stereo

Section II

Important Formulae and Constants in Optics and Their Clinical Applications

10

POWER OF LENSES

LEARNING Objectives

Upon completion of this chapter, the reader should be able to:

o calculate the power of a lens using focal length.
o calculate the focal length of a lens using power.

KEY POINTS

o Focal length (f) is the distance from the lens to the focal point where light rays either converge or appear to diverge from.
o f is expressed in meters, but may also be stated in cm or mm.
o Lens vergence (power) is expressed in diopters (D).
o f and D are inversely related and may be calculated from each other.

FOCAL LENGTH

Since plus lenses converge light (thus providing positive vergence and plus power) and minus lenses diverge light (thus providing negative vergence and minus power), the term *focal length* (f) is used to describe these characteristics. This applies to both spherical and cylindrical (minus and plus) lenses (see ahead).

The f, expressed in meters, is the distance from the lens where parallel light rays passing through a plus lens converge (Figure 10-1A) or appear to diverge from in a minus lens (Figure 10-1B). Recall that m can be converted to cm and mm, as desired.

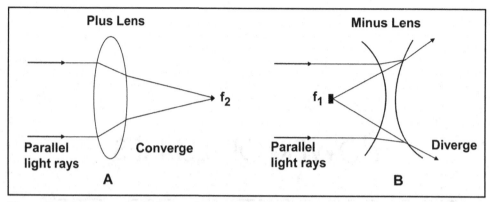

Figure 10-1: Focal length of a lens. When parallel light rays pass through a plus lens, they converge at the focal point (f_2), and the distance to that point from the lens is its focal length (A); when parallel light rays pass through a minus lens, they diverge and appear to come from its focal point (f_1), and the distance to that point from the lens is its focal length (B).

POWER OF LENSES

The power of plus and minus lenses, both spherical and cylindrical, is expressed in diopters (D), which is inversely related to f:

$$P_{(D)} = \frac{1}{f_{(m)}}$$

For the sake of convenience, cm or mm may be used instead of m, as shown below:

$$P_{(D)} = \frac{100}{f_{(cm)}} = \frac{1000}{f_{(mm)}}$$

Calculations for ophthalmic applications frequently have to determine f for a lens with a given dioptric power.

EXAMPLE 1

Calculate the power of a lens whose f is 0.3 m.

$$P_{(D)} = \frac{1}{f_{(m)}}$$

$$P_{(D)} = \frac{1}{0.3}$$

$$P_{(D)} = \frac{10}{3}$$

$$P_{(D)} = 3.33 \text{ D}$$

Note: The distance from the corneal plane to the fixation light in a Goldmann perimeter and Humphrey Field Analyzer is 30 cm. This is the reason that the basic power of a plus lens required for testing the visual field of presbyopes is +3.25 D (the value, 3.33 D, rounded off to the closest lower quarter). The actual lens used is obtained by considering +3.25 along with the refractive error and accommodative amplitude of the patient.

Example 2

Calculate the power of lenses whose fs are 200 cm, 500 mm, and 3 m.

Focal Length	Calculations for Diopter	Answers
200 cm	$P_{(D)} = \dfrac{100}{f_{(cm)}} = \dfrac{100}{200} = \dfrac{1}{2}$	0.5 D
500 mm	$P_{(D)} = \dfrac{1000}{f_{(mm)}} = \dfrac{1000}{500} = \dfrac{10}{5}$	2 D
3 m	$P_{(D)} = \dfrac{1}{f_{(m)}} = \dfrac{1}{3}$	0.33 D

The same formulae, as shown above, are used with the positions of P and f interchanged:

$$f_{(m)} = \frac{1}{P_{(D)}}$$

For the sake of convenience, cm or mm may be used instead of m, as shown below:

$$f_{(cm)} = \frac{100}{P_{(D)}} \; ; f_{(mm)} = \frac{1000}{P_{(D)}}$$

Example 3

Calculate f for a lens whose power is 2.75 D.

$$f_{(m)} = \frac{1}{P_{(D)}}$$
$$f_{(m)} = \frac{1}{2.75}$$
$$f_{(m)} = 0.36 \text{ m}$$
$$f_{(m)} = 36.4 \text{ cm}$$

Note: This is why the power of a reading add for pseudophakes is typically +2.75 D for a reading distance of approximately 36 cm. More plus power will be required to hold reading material closer, whereas less plus power will be required to hold it farther.

Example 4

Calculate the f for lenses with powers of 0.25 D, 3 D, and 5 D.

Power	Calculations for Focal Length	Answers
0.25 D	$f_{(m)} = \frac{1}{P_{(D)}} = \frac{1}{0.25}$	4 m
	$f_{(cm)} = \frac{100}{P_{(D)}} = \frac{100}{0.25}$	400 cm
	$f_{(mm)} = \frac{1000}{P_{(D)}} = \frac{1000}{0.25}$	4000 mm
3 D	$f_{(m)} = \frac{1}{P_{(D)}} = \frac{1}{3}$	0.33 m
	$f_{(cm)} = \frac{100}{P_{(D)}} = \frac{100}{3}$	33.3 cm
	$f_{(mm)} = \frac{1000}{P_{(D)}} = \frac{1000}{3}$	333.3 mm
5 D	$f_{(m)} = \frac{1}{P_{(D)}} = \frac{1}{5}$	0.2 m
	$f_{(cm)} = \frac{100}{P_{(D)}} = \frac{100}{5}$	20 cm
	$f_{(mm)} = \frac{1000}{P_{(D)}} = \frac{1000}{5}$	200 mm

Review Questions

1.   In a plus lens, the focal point is where:
     a.   total internal reflection (TIR) occurs
     b.   parallel light rays appear to diverge from
     c.   the Law of Reflection is observed
     d.   parallel light rays converge

2.   In a minus lens, the focal point is where:
     a.   TIR occurs
     b.   parallel light rays appear to diverge from
     c.   the Law of Reflection is observed
     d.   parallel light rays converge

3.   The relationship between D and f may be expressed as:
     a. $f_{(cm)} = \frac{100}{P_{(D)}}$
     b. $f_{(m)} = \frac{100}{P_{(D)}}$
     c. $P_{(D)} = \frac{100}{f_{(mm)}}$
     d. $P_{(D)} = \frac{10}{f_{(cm)}}$

4. What is the power of a lens if its f is located at 300 mm?
    a. 3 D
    b. 3.33 D
    c. 33.3 D
    d. 333 D

5. What is f for a 2.5 D lens?
    a. 400 cm
    b. 25 cm
    c. 0.4 m
    d. 2.5 m

11

VERGENCE EQUATION

LEARNING Objectives

Upon completion of this chapter, the reader should be able to:

o describe object, image, and lens vergence.
o calculate object, image, and lens vergence.

KEY POINTS

o Vergence is the ability of a lens to either converge or diverge light rays as they pass through a lens.
o Convex lenses, which converge light, are termed *plus lenses*.
o Concave lenses, which diverge light, are termed *minus lenses*.
o Parallel light rays have no vergence, and lenses are termed *plano*.
o The vergence equation states $U + P = V$ (or $U + D = V$).
o Both the vergence in diopters (U, V, and P) or distances in m, cm, or mm (u, v, or f) may be calculated.
o A lens imparts its own vergence to the incoming light—a plus lens will impart plus vergence, and a minus lens will impart minus vergence.

WHAT IS VERGENCE?

Vergence is the ability of a lens to either converge or diverge light rays as they pass through the lens (Figure 11-1).

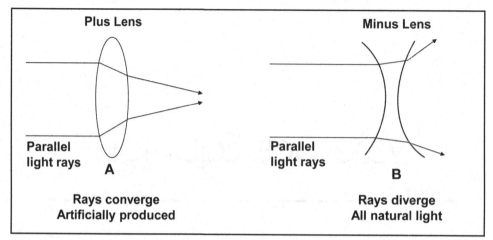

Figure 11-1. Vergence of light. In positive vergence, light converges, such as in a plus lens (A); whereas in negative vergence, light diverges, such as in a minus lens (B).

Converging light has positive vergence, and the lens that produces this effect has plus power. Convex lenses, which converge light, are therefore termed *plus lenses*. Positive vergence can only be produced by optical means such as a plus lens, and by the human eye.

Diverging light has negative vergence, and the lens that produces this effect has minus power. Concave lenses, which diverge light, are therefore termed *minus lenses*. All light—natural (eg, sunlight) and artificial (eg, lamps, flashlights and headlights)—has negative vergence. Laser light, despite being coherent and monochromatic, also has slight amounts of negative vergence.[1] Negative vergence can also be produced by optical means such as a minus lens.

Parallel light rays have no vergence, and lenses that produce this effect have no power and are termed *plano* (eg, nonprescription spectacle and contact lenses).

In clinical practice, light that travels 6 m (20 feet) or more is considered to have parallel rays and no vergence (plano power). Therefore, light that travels great distances (infinity) such as from the sun to the earth also has no vergence.

CONVENTION FOR CALCULATIONS

By convention, light is shown traveling from left to right. All distances such as focal length (f) and object and image distances are converted to diopters (D) for easy calculation.

The concepts of plus and minus space must also be applied to calculations involving the *vergence equation* (Figure 11-2). The space before light gets to the lens is termed *minus space*, whereas the space on the other side, where light emerges after passing through a lens, is termed *plus space*. Objects and images may be in either space and are assigned a plus or minus sign. Those in minus space are assigned a "–" sign, whereas those in plus space are assigned a "+" sign. That sign must be used in the calculations involving the vergence equation.

VERGENCE EQUATION

Calculations involving f and the power of a lens, and location and distance of an object and image from the lens—all with important daily clinical applications—are easily calculated using the vergence equation. Also, *object-image relationships* can be studied more easily using vergence relationships.

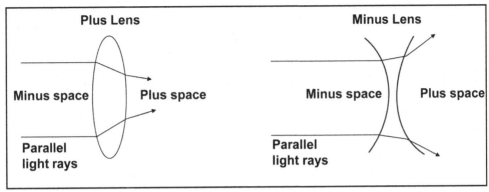

Figure 11-2. Convention for lens calculations. Light is shown traveling left to right. The area before light gets to the lens is termed minus space, whereas the area on the other side, where light emerges after passing through a lens, is termed plus space.

The vergence equation states:

$$U + P \text{ (or } D) = V$$

Where:

$U = $ object vergence (in D) $ = \frac{1}{u}$ (u is the *object distance* in m)

P or $D = $ lens vergence (in D) $ = \frac{1}{f}$ (f is the focal length in m)

$V = $ image vergence (in D) $ = \frac{1}{v}$ (v is the *image distance* in m)

Thus, vergence (in D) is simply the inverse of distance (object, focal, or image) in meters. Recall that, mathematically, D and f are inversely related and expressed as:

$$P_{(D)} = \frac{1}{f_{(m)}}$$

Recall, also, that for the sake of convenience, cm or mm may be used instead of m, as shown below:

$$P_{(D)} = \frac{100}{f_{(cm)}} = \frac{1000}{f_{(mm)}}$$

Both the vergence in D (U, V, and P) or distances in m, cm, or mm (u, v, or f) may be calculated (Table 11-1).

The vergence equation may be rearranged (see Chapter 2) in order to determine any of the three variables (Table 11-2).

Light passing through a lens will be refracted, and the amount of refraction depends on lens vergence (power of the lens). A lens imparts its own vergence to the incoming light—a plus lens will impart plus vergence, and a minus lens will impart minus vergence.

Table 11-1

Calculating Vergence[1]			
Lens vergence or power (diopters [D])	$P_{(D)} = \dfrac{1}{f_{(m)}}$	$= \dfrac{100}{f_{(cm)}}$	$= \dfrac{1000}{f_{(mm)}}$
Object vergence (D)	$U_{(D)} = \dfrac{1}{u_{(m)}}$	$= \dfrac{100}{u_{(cm)}}$	$= \dfrac{1000}{u_{(mm)}}$
Image vergence (D)	$V_{(D)} = \dfrac{1}{v_{(m)}}$	$= \dfrac{100}{v_{(cm)}}$	$= \dfrac{1000}{v_{(mm)}}$
Calculating Distance[1]			
Focal length (m, cm, or mm)	$f_{(m)} = \dfrac{1}{P_{(D)}}$ or, $f_{(cm)} = \dfrac{100}{P_{(D)}}$	or,	$f_{(mm)} = \dfrac{1000}{P_{(D)}}$
Object distance (m, cm, or mm)	$u_{(m)} = \dfrac{1}{U_{(D)}}$ or, $u_{(cm)} = \dfrac{100}{U_{(D)}}$	or,	$u_{(mm)} = \dfrac{1000}{U_{(D)}}$
Image distance (m, cm, or mm)	$v_{(m)} = \dfrac{1}{V_{(D)}}$ or, $v_{(cm)} = \dfrac{100}{V_{(D)}}$	or,	$v_{(mm)} = \dfrac{1000}{V_{(D)}}$

[1]Also see Chapter 10.

Table 11-2

Vergence Equation: $U + P = V$	
Variable	**Equation**
Image vergence (V)	$V = U + P$
Object vergence (U)	$U = V - P$
Lens vergence, or power (P)	$P = V - U$

CALCULATIONS

Since the area before light gets to a lens is termed minus space, light originating from an object is divergent and has negative vergence (see Figure 11-2). Therefore, a minus sign is assigned to object vergence in all calculations involving single lenses, making the vergence equation $-U + P = V$. In an array of multiple lenses, however, U may be plus or minus depending on the location of the object. Please see Chapter 12 for more details.

Light passing through a lens will form an image, and the light rays will also have some vergence. The position of the image depends on lens power and the distance of the object from the lens, as depicted in the vergence equation. Remember, vergence variables (U, P, and V) are expressed in D and may be calculated using m, cm, or mm.

The only equations you need to recall are shown below:

Calculating image vergence (V): $V = U + P$
Calculating object vergence (U): $U = V - P$
Calculating lens vergence (P): $P = V - U$

Recall that the space before light gets to the lens is termed *minus space*, whereas the space on the other side, where light emerges after passing through a lens, is termed *plus space*. Objects and images may be in either space and are assigned a "–" or "+" sign based on their location. This sign must be used in the calculations involving the vergence equation.

Using the appropriate equation, vergence calculations are completed in 3 steps:

1. Convert u, f, or v (m, cm, or mm) to D.
2. Calculate missing variable (U, P, or V) using equation.
3. Convert U, P, or V (D) to m, cm, or mm.

Example 1

An object is 2000 mm in front of a +4.50 D lens. Where is the image located?

Object distance (u): 2000 mm

Object vergence ($U_{(D)}$): $U_{(D)} = \dfrac{1000}{u_{(mm)}}$

$$U_{(D)} = \dfrac{1000}{2000}$$

$$U_{(D)} = \dfrac{1}{2}$$

$$U_{(D)} = 0.5\ D$$

Vergence equation: $V = U + P$
$U = 0.5\ D, P = +4.50\ D$

Since object vergence is negative, the vergence equation becomes:
$$V = -U + P$$

Substituting values (parentheses are used just for convenience):
$$V = (-0.5) + (+4.50)$$
$$V = -0.5 + 4.50$$
$$V = +4\ D$$

Thus, the image vergence is +4 D. The "+" sign indicates that the image is in plus space.

Now, calculate the image distance based on a vergence of +4 D. We can calculate this distance in m, cm, or mm. Since the object distance was stated in mm, we can calculate the image distance in mm.

Image distance: $v_{(mm)} = \dfrac{1000}{V_{(D)}}$

$$v_{(mm)} = \dfrac{1000}{4}$$

$$v_{(mm)} = 250\ mm$$

Thus, the image of an object 2000 mm in front of a +4.50 D lens is located in plus space and 250 mm from the lens.

Example 2

An image forms 100 cm behind a lens when an object is 500 mm in front of it. What is the power of the lens?

Object distance (u):   500 mm

Object vergence ($U_{(D)}$): $U_{(D)} = \dfrac{1000}{u_{(mm)}}$

$U_{(D)} = \dfrac{1000}{500}$

$U_{(D)} = 2\ D$

Image distance (v):   100 cm

Image vergence ($V_{(D)}$): $V_{(D)} = \dfrac{100}{v_{(cm)}}$

$V_{(D)} = \dfrac{100}{100}$

$V_{(D)} = \dfrac{1}{1}$

$V_{(D)} = 1\ D$

Vergence equation: $V = U + P$

$U = 2\ D,\ V = 1\ D$

The vergence equation has to be rearranged for P:

$P = V - U$

Since object vergence is negative, the vergence equation becomes:

$P = V - (-U)$

Substituting values (parentheses are used just for convenience):

$P = (1) - (-2)$

$P = 1 + 2$

$P = +3\ D$

Thus, the power of the lens that forms an image 100 cm behind it when an object is 500 mm in front of it is +3 D.

Example 3

Calculate the image vergence and image location of an object held 0.075 m in front of a +90 D lens (NOTE: 1 m = 100 cm = 1000 mm).

Object vergence (in D): $U = \dfrac{1}{u}$ (u is the object distance in m)

$U = \dfrac{1}{0.075}$

$U = 13.3\ D$

Image vergence (V) may now be calculated. Note that a minus sign is used for U in this example:

$V = U + P$

$V = -(+13.3) + (+90)$

$V = -13.3 + 90$

$V = +76.7\ D$

The plus sign in front of 76.7 D indicates that the image forms on the other side of the lens from the object.

Image vergence, V (+76.7 D), may be converted to image distance (image location):

Image distance in m (v) $= \frac{1}{V}$ (V = image vergence [in D])

Image distance in m (v) $= \frac{1}{76.7}$

$$v = 0.013 \text{ m}$$
$$v = 1.3 \text{ cm}$$

This is the reason that, during a dilated fundus examination, a +90 D lens is held approximately 5 cm from the eye, and the slit lamp beam is focused at approximately 1.3 cm from the +90 D lens in order to observe the fundus image.

Reference

1. Thall EH, Miller KM, Rosenthal P, Schechter RJ, Steinert RF, Beardsley TL. *Basic and Clinical Science Course, Section 3: Optics, Refraction, and Contact Lenses.* San Francisco, CA: American Academy of Ophthalmology; 2000.

Review Questions

1. The vergence equation may be rewritten as:
    a. $V + P = U$
    b. $U - V = P$
    c. $V - P = U$
    d. $U - P = V$

2. Vergences can be converted to D by using the following formula:
    a. $D = \text{distance}_{(m)}$
    b. $\text{distance}_{(m)} = \frac{D}{1}$
    c. $D = \frac{1}{\text{distance}_{(m)}}$
    d. $D = \frac{\text{distance}_{(m)}}{1}$

3. The object vergence of a candle placed at 50 m from a lens is:
    a.   0.2 D
    b.   0.02 D
    c.   5.0 D
    d.   2 D

4. What is the power of the lens if an image forms 2 m in plus space when an object is 500 mm in front of it?
    a.   +2.5 D
    b.   +2.00 D
    c.   −2.5 D
    d.   +1.5 D

5.   An object is 400 cm in front of a –2.75 D lens. Where is the image located?
        a.   –4.00 D
        b.   33.3 cm in plus space
        c.   +4.00 D
        d.   33.3 cm in minus space

12

Multiple Lens Systems

Learning Objectives

Upon completion of this chapter, the reader should be able to:

o describe object, image, and lens vergence in multiple lens systems.
o calculate object, image, and lens vergence in multiple lens systems.

Key Points

o The vergence equation may be used to calculate the location of the final image in a multiple lens system.
o The image formed by the first lens becomes the object for the second lens, and the image formed by the second lens becomes the object for the third lens, and so on.
o The vergence equation is applied independently to each lens in the system.
o The image vergence provided by the final lens in the system is the location of the final image produced by the entire multiple lens system.
o Since the image of the first lens becomes the object for the second lens, this object might be present in plus space or minus space of the second lens, and a "+" or "−" sign, respectively, must be assigned to U for the second lens.

VERGENCE EQUATION

The vergence equation may be used to calculate the location of the *final image* in a *multiple lens system*. The vergence equation states:

$$U + P \text{ (or } D) = V$$

Note: For details of vergence, vergence equation, and vergence calculations, see Chapter 11.

Since all light rays are divergent, a minus sign is assigned to object vergence in all calculations involving single lenses, thus making the vergence equation $-U + P = V$. In an array of multiple lenses, however, U may be plus or minus depending on the location of the object (see ahead).

MULTIPLE LENS SYSTEMS

Many ophthalmic and optical lenses are actually multiple lens systems in which each lens imparts its vergence to light rays such that the final image is appropriately produced. The most familiar example of this is the lens of a digital or SLR camera, including telephoto lenses. A complex system of lenses actually comprises the lens. Increasingly common ophthalmic examples are *piggyback lenses*. *Aphakic* patients are frequently given a soft contact lens on the cornea with a rigid gas-permeable (RGP) lens riding piggyback on the soft lens. High myopes are frequently given implants of a phakic intraocular lens (IOL) that rides piggyback on the natural crystalline lens.

While ophthalmic medical personnel (OMP) do not routinely have to make calculations for multiple lens systems, knowing how to do this is an added professional skill that can be used to assist ophthalmologists and patients.

In multiple lens systems, the image formed by the first lens becomes the object for the second lens, and the image formed by the second lens becomes the object for the third lens, and so on.

The vergence equation is applied independently to each lens in the system. The image vergence provided by the final lens in the system is the location of the final image produced by the entire multiple lens system.

Remember to assign the proper algebraic sign to the object and image vergence. Since the image of the first lens becomes the object for the second lens, this object might be present in plus space or minus space of the second lens and a "+" or "–" sign, respectively, must be assigned to U (object vergence) for the second lens.

In the same way, determine whether the object for the next lens in the system is present in plus or minus space for that lens.

EXAMPLE 1

Where will the final image form if an object is placed 50 mm in front of a +10.00 D lens that is separated from a +5.00 D lens by 100 cm?

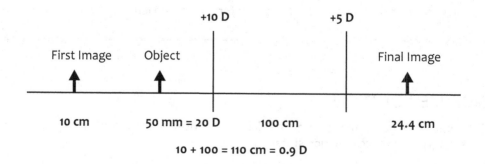

First Lens	Second Lens
$U + P = V$	$U + P = V$
$(-20) + (+10) = V$	$(-0.9) + (+5) = V$
$-20 + 10 = V$	$-0.9 + 5 = V$
$-10\ D = V$	$+4.1\ D = V$
$f_{(cm)} = \frac{100}{10} = 10$ cm	$f_{(cm)} = \frac{100}{4.1} = 24.4$ cm
First image= 10 cm	Final image = 24.4 cm

Example 2

Where will the final image form if an object is placed 50 m in front of a –1.00 D lens that is separated from a –3.00 D lens by 10 cm?

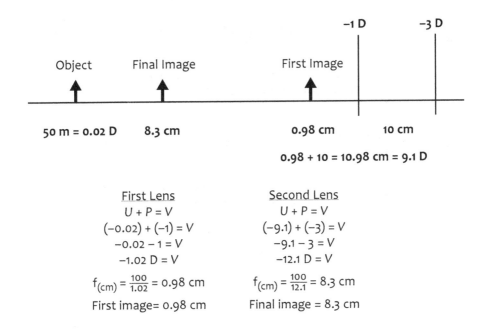

0.98 + 10 = 10.98 cm = 9.1 D

First Lens	Second Lens
$U + P = V$	$U + P = V$
$(-0.02) + (-1) = V$	$(-9.1) + (-3) = V$
$-0.02 - 1 = V$	$-9.1 - 3 = V$
$-1.02\ D = V$	$-12.1\ D = V$
$f_{(cm)} = \frac{100}{1.02} = 0.98$ cm	$f_{(cm)} = \frac{100}{12.1} = 8.3$ cm
First image= 0.98 cm	Final image = 8.3 cm

Review Questions

1. Where will the final image form if an object is placed 500 mm in front of a –2.00 D lens that is separated from a +5.00 D lens by 25 cm?
    a. 25 cm from the final lens and in its minus space
    b. 33.3 cm from the final lens and in its minus space
    c. 25 cm from the final lens and in its plus space
    d. 33.3 cm from the final lens and in its plus space

2. Where will the final image form if an object is placed at infinity in front of a +10.00 D lens that is separated from a +1.00 D lens by 110 cm?
    a. 10 cm from the plus lens and in its plus space
    b. at infinity in the plus space of the +1.00 lens
    c. 10 cm from the plus lens and in its minus space
    d. 1 m from the plus lens and in its minus space

3. What is the location of the final image if an object is placed 10 cm before a +10 D lens that is separated from another +10 D lens?
    a. 10 cm from the second lens and in its plus space
    b. 10 m from the second lens and in its plus space
    c. 10 cm from the second lens and in its minus space
    d. at infinity in plus space of the first lens

4. What is the location of the final image if an object is placed 10 cm before a +10 D lens that is separated from a –2 D lens?
    a. 25 cm from the minus lens and in its plus space
    b. 50 cm from the minus lens and in its plus space
    c. 25 cm from the minus lens and in its minus space
    d. 50 cm from the minus lens and in its minus space

5. What is the location of the final image if rays from infinity travel through a –5 D lens that is separated by 80 cm from a –3 D lens?
    a. 25 cm from the first lens and in its plus space
    b. 25 cm from the second lens and in its minus space
    c. 20 cm from the first lens and in its plus space
    d. 20 cm from the second lens and in its minus space

13

MAGNIFICATION BY LENSES

LEARNING Objectives

Upon completion of this chapter, the reader should be able to:

o   describe magnification and reduction of lens images.
o   calculate magnification by lenses.

KEY POINTS

o   Magnification refers to the magnification produced by a plus lens and reduction produced by a minus lens.
o   Magnification may be calculated using object and image distances or sizes.
o   Magnification $= \dfrac{\text{image distance}}{\text{object distance}}$
o   Magnification $= \dfrac{\text{image size}}{\text{object size}}$

MAGNIFICATION

Even though the term *magnification* is used for image size and implies "enlargement" of an image, the term is used for both magnification produced by a plus lens and reduction produced by a minus lens.[1]

There are many ways to describe and calculate magnification produced by lenses:

o   Magnification calculated from the *object* and *image distances* from the lens
o   Magnification calculated from the *object* and *image sizes*

CALCULATING MAGNIFICATION USING DISTANCES

Magnification is determined by comparing the image distance to the object distance (Figure 13-1):

$$\text{Magnification} = \frac{\text{Image distance}}{\text{Object distance}}$$

o   Images produced by plus lenses are located in plus space and are inverted.

o   Images produced by minus lenses are located in minus space and are upright.

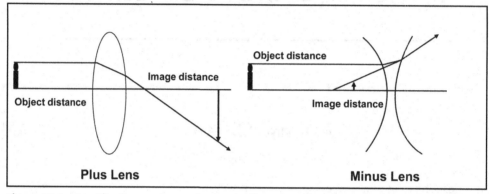

Figure 13-1. Magnification compares the image distance to the object distance. In plus lenses, images are located in plus space and are inverted; whereas in minus lenses, images are located in minus space and are upright.

CALCULATING MAGNIFICATION USING SIZES

Magnification is also calculated by comparing image size to object size. Images twice as large have a magnification of 2, whereas images half as large have a magnification of 0.5.

$$\text{Magnification} = \frac{\text{Image size}}{\text{Object size}}$$

CALCULATIONS

The formulae shown above may be used for calculating any of the variables.

EXAMPLE 1

What is the magnification of the image produced by a +2.5 D lens if an object is placed 2 m from the lens and in its minus space?

$$
\begin{aligned}
\text{Object distance } (u) &= 2 \text{ m} \\
\text{Object vergence } (U) &= \tfrac{1}{2} \\
U &= 0.5 \text{ D} \\
\text{Power of lens } (P) &= +2.5 \text{ D} \\
\text{Vergence equation} &= V = U + P \\
\text{Image vergence } (V) &= (-0.5) + (+2.5) \\
V &= -0.5 + 2.5 \\
V &= +2 \text{ D}
\end{aligned}
$$

$$\text{Image distance} = \frac{1}{V}$$
$$= \frac{1}{2}$$
$$= 0.5 \text{ m}$$
$$\text{Magnification} = \frac{\text{Image distance}}{\text{Object distance}}$$
$$= \frac{0.5}{2}$$
$$= \frac{5}{20}$$
$$= \frac{1}{4}$$
$$= 0.25$$

The image will be ¼ the size of the object.

Example 2

What is the magnification of the image produced by a –1.5 D lens if an object is placed 2 m from the lens and in its minus space?

$$\text{Object distance } (u) = 2 \text{ m}$$
$$\text{Object vergence } (U) = \frac{1}{2}$$
$$U = 0.5 \text{ D}$$
$$\text{Power of lens } (P) = -1.5 \text{ D}$$
$$\text{Vergence equation} = V = U + P$$
$$\text{Image vergence } (V) = (-0.5) + (-1.5)$$
$$V = -0.5 - 1.5$$
$$V = -2 \text{ D}$$
$$\text{Image distance} = \frac{1}{V}$$
$$= \frac{1}{2}$$
$$= 0.5 \text{ m}$$
$$\text{Magnification} = \frac{\text{Image distance}}{\text{Object distance}}$$
$$= \frac{0.5}{2}$$
$$= \frac{5}{20}$$
$$= \frac{1}{4}$$
$$= 0.25$$

The image will be ¼ the size of the object.

Example 3

What is the magnification if a plus lens creates a 20-cm-tall image of a 4-cm-tall object?

$$\text{Object size} = 4 \text{ cm}$$
$$\text{Image size} = 20 \text{ cm}$$
$$\text{Magnification} = \frac{\text{Image size}}{\text{Object size}}$$

$$= \frac{20}{4}$$

$$= 5$$

The image will be 5 times the size of the object.

References

1. Thall EH, Miller KM, Rosenthal P, Schechter RJ, Steinert RF, Beardsley TL. *Basic and Clinical Science Course, Section 3: Optics, Refraction, and Contact Lenses*. San Francisco, CA: American Academy of Ophthalmology; 2000.

Review Questions

1. What is the magnification of the image produced by a +2 D lens if an object is placed 1 m from the lens and in its minus space?
   a. 1
   b. 2
   c. 3
   d. 4

2. What is the magnification of the image produced by a –1.5 D lens if an object is placed 2 m from the lens and in its minus space?
   a. 2.5
   b. 0.5
   c. 0.25
   d. 5.0

3. What is the magnification if a plus lens creates a 10-cm-tall image of a 2-cm-tall object?
   a. 2
   b. 5
   c. 10
   d. 20

4. How tall is the image produced by a plus lens that magnifies a 5-cm-tall object 10 times?
   a. 10 cm
   b. 5 cm
   c. 50 cm
   d. 2 cm

5. How tall is the object if a minus lens produces its image 10 cm tall and magnified 0.5 times?

    a.   2 cm
    b.   5 cm
    c.   10 cm
    d.   20 cm

14

PRISMS AND DISPERSION

LEARNING Objectives

Upon completion of this chapter, the reader should be able to:

o   calculate power of prisms and displacement of images.
o   describe breakup of white light into its component colors.

KEY POINTS

o   Prisms have an apex and a base, and bend light toward the prism base.
o   The greater the apex angle, the greater the prismatic effect.
o   Two types of images are produced by prisms: real and virtual.
o   The power of a prism is measured in prism diopter (PD or $^\Delta$).
o   1 PD or 1^Δ displaces the real image by 1 cm at a distance of 1 m from the prism.
o   White light passing through a prism separates into its component colors.
o   The sequence of colors is termed a *spectrum*, and the phenomenon is termed *dispersion*.
o   Colors are dispersed by different amounts depending on the wavelength of the color.
o   Blue has the shortest wavelength (greatest frequency) and disperses the most.
o   Red has the longest wavelength (lowest frequency) and disperses the least.

PRISM MORPHOLOGY

A prism is a wedge-shaped refracting medium whose surfaces are at an angle to each other (ie, not parallel). Prisms have an apex and a base, and light is refracted according to Snell's law and bends toward the prism base (Figure 14-1).

The prismatic effect (ie, *light rays bending* and displacement of the real image toward the prism base) is determined by the apex angle between the two refracting surfaces. The greater the apex angle, the greater the prismatic effect (Figure 14-2).

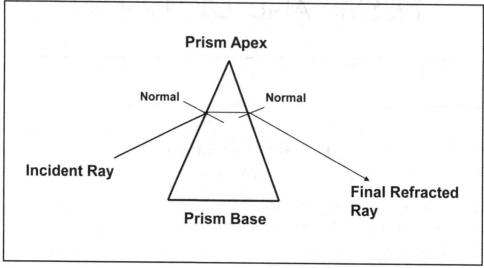

Figure 14-1. Refraction by a prism. Light is refracted by both surfaces of a prism in accordance with Snell's Law. The first refracted ray, inside the prism, bends toward the normal, whereas the final refracted ray bends away from the normal. Thus, all light rays emerging from the prism bend toward the prism base.

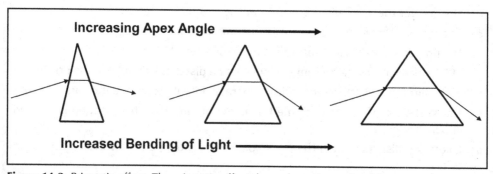

Figure 14-2. Prismatic effect. The prismatic effect depends on the angle of the apex. The greater the angle, the greater the bending of light toward the prism base.

PRISM IMAGES

There are two types of *prism images* (Figure 14-3). When light shines through a prism, the image produced by the bending of light toward the base is termed the *real image* because it can form on a screen held on the other side of the prism from the light source (Figure 14-3A). This image has anatomical significance because it may be moved to a different place on the retina by including prism in one or both spectacle lenses for eliminating *diplopia*. When light bends toward the *spectacle lens prism base*, the real image on the retina is moved on the fovea from a different place, thus producing fusion and eliminating diplopia.

On the other hand, if the object is viewed through the prism, it will appear to be displaced toward the apex. This image is termed *virtual* because it cannot form on a screen held on the other side of the prism from the object (Figure 14-3B).

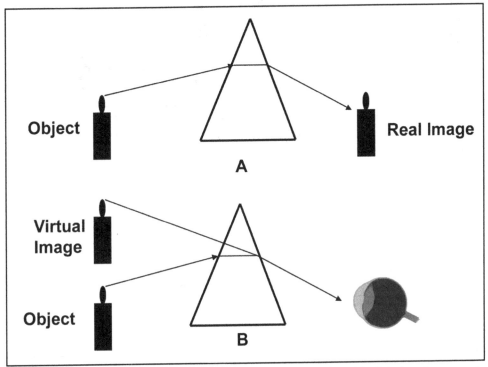

Figure 14-3. Images produced by a prism. The real image is produced by light bending toward the prism base (A). The virtual image appears displaced toward the prism apex when the object is viewed through the prism (B).

PRISM POWER

The power of a prism is its ability to bend light and displace the real image toward the prism base. *Prism power* is measured in *prism diopters*, which is abbreviated as "PD" or with a superscript triangle ($^\Delta$) (Figure 14-4).

1 PD or 1^Δ displaces the real image toward the prism base by 1 cm at a distance of 1 m from the prism.

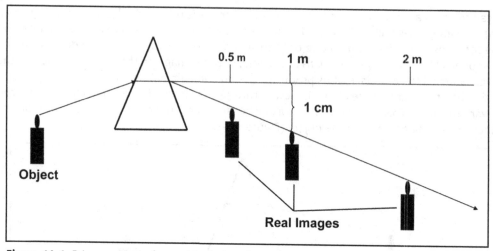

Figure 14-4. Prism power is denoted in "prism diopter" (abbreviated as PD or by a superscript triangle [$^\Delta$]) and denotes real image displacement toward the prism base at a distance of 1 m. 1 PD (1^Δ) displaces the real image by 1 cm at a distance of 1 m.

Expressed mathematically (Figure 14-5):

$$P = \frac{C}{D}$$

Where:
P =   prism power (PD or $^\Delta$)
C =   displacement of real image toward prism base (cm)
D =   distance of real image from prism (m)

Note: The unit for the real image displacement is cm, but it is usually denoted in mm and must be converted to cm. See Chapter 1 for details.

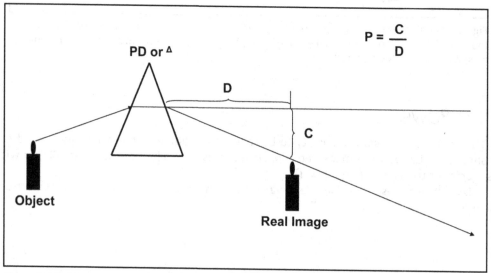

Figure 14-5. Prism power is denoted in "prism diopter" (abbreviated as "PD" or by a superscript triangle [$^\Delta$]) and is equal to $\frac{C}{D}$.

A few useful rules may be summarized relating to prism power and displacement of the real image toward the prism base:

- o Prism power < 1^Δ = displaces a real image < 1 cm toward prism base at 1 m from the prism
- o Prism power > 1^Δ = displaces a real image > 1 cm toward prism base at 1 m from the prism

In any prism, the real image will appear to be displaced more toward the prism base if the screen is farther from the prism:

1^Δ =   displaces a real image 1 cm toward prism base at 1 m from the prism
1^Δ =   displaces a real image 2 cm toward prism base at 2 m from the prism
1^Δ =   displaces a real image 5 cm toward prism base at 5 m from the prism

CALCULATIONS

Any of the three variables (P, D, or C) may be calculated either by drawing a sketch (see Figure 14-4) to determine the unknown variable, or by using the formula (see Figure 14-5). If the formula is used, it will have to be rearranged in order to calculate C or D (Table 14-1).

Table 14-1	
Variable	**Formula[1]**
Power of prism (PD or Δ)	$P = \dfrac{C}{D}$
Displacement of real image toward prism base (cm)	$C = (P)\,(D)$
Distance of real image from prism (m)	$D = \dfrac{C}{P}$

[1]P is denoted in prism diopter, C in cm, and D in m.

EXAMPLE 1

How far is the real image displaced by a 5^Δ at a distance of 50 cm?

$$P \;=\; 5^\Delta$$
$$D \;=\; 50 \text{ cm}$$
$$D \;=\; \frac{50}{100}$$
$$D \;=\; \frac{5}{10}$$
$$D \;=\; \frac{1}{2}$$
$$D \;=\; 0.5 \text{ m}$$
$$C \;=\; (P)\,(D)$$
$$C \;=\; (5)\,(0.5)$$
$$C \;=\; 2.5 \text{ cm}$$

A 5^Δ prism will displace a real image 2.5 cm toward its base at a distance of 50 cm.

Example 2

What is the power of a prism that displaces a real image 4 cm toward the base at a distance of 200 cm?

$$C = 4 \text{ cm}$$
$$D = 200 \text{ cm}$$
$$D = \frac{200}{100}$$
$$D = \frac{2}{1}$$
$$D = 2 \text{ m}$$
$$P = \frac{C}{D}$$
$$P = \frac{4}{2}$$
$$P = 2^\Delta$$

The power of a prism that displaces a real image 4 cm toward its base at a distance of 200 cm is 2^Δ.

Example 3

How far from a 3^Δ prism will a real image be displaced 60 mm toward the prism base?

$$P = 3^\Delta$$
$$C = 60 \text{ mm}$$
$$C = \frac{60}{10}$$
$$C = \frac{6}{1}$$
$$C = 6 \text{ cm}$$
$$D = \frac{C}{P}$$
$$D = \frac{6}{3}$$
$$D = 2 \text{ m}$$

A real image will be displaced 60 mm toward the prism base by a 3^Δ prism at a distance of 2 m from the prism.

CLINICAL USES OF PRISMS

Prisms have many clinical uses in ophthalmology:
- Measurements of muscle imbalances. Prisms displace the real image, moving it on the fovea of the deviated eye, thus producing fusion and eliminating corrective eye movements on cover testing.
- A prism determined by cover testing is incorporated into one or both spectacle lenses to eliminate fusion difficulties and diplopia.
- *Base out prisms* for eye exercises to correct *convergence insufficiency*.
- Ophthalmic instruments such as *Goldmann applanation tonometer*, exophthalmometer, ophthalmometer (Keratometer), corneal alignment device, and *Risley prism* on the refractor (Phoroptor).

o   Optical instruments such as binoculars, *Fresnel searchlights*, and plastic *Fresnel prisms* to affix on spectacle lenses.

DISPERSION

Sir Isaac Newton demonstrated that white light passing through a prism separates into its component colors. Newton termed the sequence of colors a *spectrum* and the phenomenon *dispersion*. *Rainbows* and colors produced by oil are examples of dispersion.

The order of colors from the prism base toward the prism apex is always the same (Figure 14-6). This sequence may be easily recalled by the mnemonics VIBGYOR or ROYGBIV.

Prism base: Violet
Indigo
Blue
Green
Yellow
Orange
Prism apex: Red

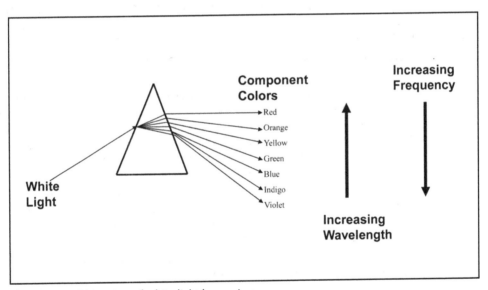

Figure 14-6. Dispersion of white light by a prism.

During dispersion, colors are refracted and dispersed by different amounts depending on the wavelength of the color. (NOTE: Frequency may be stated instead of wavelength, and both are inversely related.)

o   Blue has the shortest wavelength (greatest frequency), disperses the most, and appears toward the prism base.

o   Red has the longest wavelength (lowest frequency), disperses the least, and appears toward the prism apex.

CLINICAL USES OF COLORED LIGHT

Colors (think wavelengths and frequencies of VIBGYOR) have many clinical uses in ophthalmology.

FLUORESCEIN

(See Fluorescence in Chapter 3.)

Fluorescein sodium dye is one of the most commonly used pharmacologic agents in ophthalmology. An *orange dye*, fluorescein sodium, is supplied on a filter paper or in 5 mL or 10 mL bottles. When the orange color of fluorescein is stimulated by blue light using a *cobalt blue filter*, green fluorescence is produced and may be observed using a slit lamp (biomicroscope), tonometer, direct *ophthalmoscope*, or a fundus camera. Many practitioners use a yellow *Wratten filter* to block reflected cobalt blue light, thus allowing a better visualization of the green fluorescence.

As described in Chapter 3, the *fluorescent wavelength* (green) is longer than the *excitation wavelength* (blue).

Fluorescein has important uses in ophthalmic procedures:

o The corneal epithelium prevents the corneal stroma from absorbing fluorescein, and no fluorescein staining is seen in a slit lamp examination if the epithelium is intact. However, in corneal erosions, abrasions, ulcers, and *Herpes simplex* dendritic lesions, the epithelial cells are damaged and the epithelium may be absent. This allows the stroma to absorb fluorescein, which appears as bright green areas during a slit lamp examination.

o *Semicircular green mires* are used in Goldmann applanation tonometry to obtain intraocular pressure.

o Fluorescein angiography is used to evaluate whether retinal arteries, veins, and neovascular growths are intact or leak serum. Five mL of 10% fluorescein sodium is injected intravenously after the patient with dilated eyes is properly positioned at the fundus camera. Within 8 to 10 seconds, the fluorescein appears in the eye and photos are obtained to determine areas of leakage. These areas may be photocoagulated with an argon laser. As an alternative to intravenous administration, a patient apprehensive of the injection may be given oral fluorescein with a fruit drink. In this case, the waiting period is greater, and the patient must be continuously monitored in order to obtain the earliest set of photos as fluorescein enters the eye, which is the most useful set.

o In a slit lamp examination, an even spread of fluorescein under a rigid gas-permeable (RGP) contact lens indicates a good RGP fit. On the other hand, central pooling with excessive peripheral touch indicates a steep-fitting RPG, whereas peripheral pooling with a central touch indicates a flat-fitting RGP. Many RGP fitters insert a yellow Wratten filter, which blocks reflected cobalt blue light and allows a better visualization of the green fluorescence.

o After small-incision *extracapsular cataract extraction* by *phacoemulsification*, the small surgical incision is evaluated to check for leakage using fluorescein and to determine whether a surgical suture should be used. A sterile fluorescein strip is touched on the surgical incision. An incision that has closed well will not leak or might only leak minor amounts of aqueous, whereas an open incision will leak greater amounts of aqueous and a green rivulet will flow out from the incision (positive *Seidel test*), indicating that a suture might be needed.[1]

Red-Free Light

In ophthalmic practice, green light is termed *red-free light*, and this wavelength is absorbed by red blood cells. Therefore, the red-free setting on a slit lamp is used to examine conjunctival, episcleral, and scleral vasculature in order to distinguish between conjunctivitis (of which there are many kinds), episcleritis, and scleritis.

REFERENCE

1. Kunimoto DY, Kanitkar KD, Makar MS. *The Wills Eye Manual: Office and Emergency Room Diagnosis and Treatment of Eye Diseases.* New York, NY: Lippincott Williams & Wilkins; 2004.

REVIEW QUESTIONS

1. What is the real image displacement at 2 m by a 2^Δ prism?
    - a.   2 cm
    - b.   4 mm
    - c.   2 mm
    - d.   4 cm

2. What is the real image displacement at 1 km in a 0.5^Δ prism?
    - a.   500 cm
    - b.   5 cm
    - c.   5 km
    - d.   500 km

3. How far from a 10^Δ prism is a real image if it is displaced 100 mm?
    - a.   10 m
    - b.   1 m
    - c.   10 cm
    - d.   10 mm

4. What is the power of a prism that displaces a real image 5 mm at 2 m?
    - a. 2.5^Δ
    - b. 0.25^Δ
    - c. 25^Δ
    - d. 0.025^Δ

5. What is the power of a prism that displaces a real image 100 cm at 1 km?
    - a. 1^Δ
    - b. 10^Δ
    - c. 0.01^Δ
    - d. 0.1^Δ

15

POWER OF MIRRORS

LEARNING OBJECTIVES

Upon completion of this chapter, the reader should be able to:

o   describe the power of concave and convex mirrors.
o   calculate the power of concave and convex mirrors.

KEY POINTS

o   Parallel rays striking a concave mirror are reflected back, passing through the center of curvature.
o   Parallel rays striking a convex mirror are reflected back and appear to originate from the center of curvature.
o   Reflecting power of concave and convex mirrors is expressed in diopters (D), which is the inverse of the focal length (f) (in m) of the mirror.
o   The f (in m) of a mirror is half the radius of curvature (r) of the mirror.

CONVENTION FOR CALCULATIONS

Just as in lenses, light is shown traveling from left to right. Other conventions, however, differ from those of lenses (Figure 15-1):

o   The chief ray of mirrors passes through the center of curvature and is reflected back in the same direction.
o   Parallel rays striking a concave mirror are reflected back so they pass through the center of curvature.

o Parallel rays striking a convex mirror are reflected back so they appear to originate from the center of curvature.

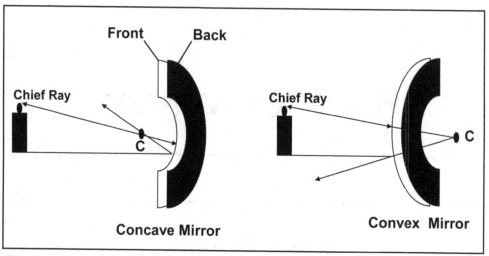

Figure 15-1. Nomenclature for mirrors. The chief ray of mirrors passes through the center of curvature (C) and is reflected back in the same direction. Parallel rays striking a concave mirror are reflected back so they pass through the center of curvature. Parallel rays striking a convex mirror are reflected back so they appear to originate from the center of curvature.

POWER OF MIRRORS

Reflecting power of concave and convex mirrors is expressed in diopters (D) and is the inverse of the focal length (*f*) (in m) of the mirror:

$$D = \frac{1}{f}$$

Where:
   D = reflecting *power of a mirror* in D
   f = focal length of a mirror in m

According to convention, the *f* (in m) of a mirror is half the *radius of curvature* (r) of the mirror.

$$f = \frac{r}{2}$$

Where:
   r = radius of curvature of a mirror in m

Thus (Figure 15-2),

$$D = \frac{1}{f} = \frac{2}{r}$$

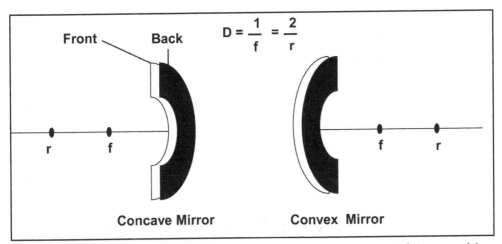

Figure 15-2. Reflecting power of convex and concave mirrors in diopters (D) is the inverse of the focal length (*f*), which is equal to half the radius of curvature (*r*) of the mirror.

Example 1

What is the power of a mirror whose *f* is 25 cm?

$$D = \frac{1}{f}$$
$$D = \frac{1}{0.25}$$
$$D = 4\ D$$

Example 2

What is the power of a mirror whose *r* is 50 cm?

$$D = \frac{2}{r}$$
$$D = \frac{2}{0.5}$$
$$D = 4\ D$$

Example 3

What is the *f* in cm of a mirror whose power is 5 D?

$$D = \frac{1}{f}$$
$$f = \frac{1}{D}$$
$$f = \frac{1}{5}$$
$$f = 0.2\ m$$
$$f = 20\ cm$$

Example 4

What is the r in cm of a mirror whose power is 2 D?

$$D = \frac{2}{r}$$
$$r = \frac{2}{D}$$
$$r = \frac{2}{2}$$
$$r = 1\,m$$
$$r = 100\,cm$$

Review Questions

1. The power and r of a mirror may be mathematically related as:
    - a.   (D) (3) = r
    - b.   (D) (r) = 2
    - c.   D = (2) (r)
    - d.   (D) (2) = r

2. The f and r of a mirror may be mathematically related as:
    - a. $r = \frac{2}{f}$
    - b. $f = 2r$
    - c. $f = \frac{2}{r}$
    - d. $r = 2f$

3. What is the power of a mirror whose f is 33 cm?
    - a.   2 D
    - b.   3 D
    - c.   4 D
    - d.   5 D

4. What is the power of a mirror whose r is 250 mm?
    - a.   7 D
    - b.   8 D
    - c.   9 D
    - d.   10 D

5. What is the f of a mirror whose power is 2 D?
    - a.   50 cm
    - b.   5 m
    - c.   50 m
    - d.   5 cm

16

SPHERICAL LENSES

LEARNING OBJECTIVES

Upon completion of this chapter, the reader should be able to:

o   describe the power of spherical lenses.
o   describe spherical lens prescriptions.

KEY POINTS

o   Spherical lenses have spherical curved surfaces and the same power in all meridians.
o   Spherical lenses can be minus or plus, and are used to correct myopia and hyperopia.
o   Plus power of myopic eyes is decreased by using minus lenses.
o   Plus power of hyperopic eyes is increased by using plus lenses.

SPHERICAL LENS

Spherical (usually shortened to sphere) lenses have spherical curved surfaces and, therefore, the same power in all meridians. In clinical applications, the terms *axis* and *meridian* are frequently used interchangeably.

Since the power is the same in every meridian of a spherical lens, light rays will have the same vergence (ie, in a plus lens, all light rays will converge equally, whereas in a minus lens, all light rays will diverge equally).

Because light rays in spherical lenses either converge or diverge equally, images produced by spherical lenses form a point focus at the focal point of the spherical lens.

The image produced by a plus spherical lens forms a point focus (focal point) in the plus space of the lens, where all light rays eventually converge (Figure 16-1A). The image produced by a minus spherical lens appears to come from a point focus in the minus space of the lens, from where all light rays appear to diverge (Figure 16-1B) (see Chapters 8 and 11).

Images formed by spherical lenses in this way are termed *stigmatic images*.

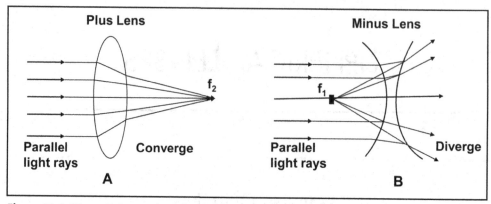

Figure 16-1. Stigmatic images by spherical lenses. Light rays in spherical lenses either converge or diverge equally, and images produced by spherical lenses form a point focus at the focal point of the spherical lens. The image produced by a plus spherical lens forms in the plus space of the lens (f_2) where all light rays converge (A). The image produced by a minus spherical lens appears to come from minus space of the lens (f_1) from where all light rays appear to diverge (B).

Spherical lenses therefore only have one parameter—power. Such lenses can be plus or minus, and will display characteristics of those lenses (eg, image movement, magnification, central and peripheral thickness, etc) (see Chapters 8 and 11).

Concepts of speed of light, refractive index (RI), Snell's law, bending of light across an interface with two different RI, critical angle (i_c), total internal reflection (TIR), and prismatic nature of lenses described so far all apply to spherical lenses.

Focal length (f), diopters (D), vergence, and magnification may be calculated for spherical lenses using the formulae described in earlier chapters.

CORRECTION OF REFRACTIVE ERRORS (LENS PRESCRIPTIONS)

(Also see Chapters 21, 22, and 24.)

When light rays enter the human eye, the sum of all refraction by the tears, cornea, aqueous, lens, and vitreous results in plus vergence (convergence). Thus, the human eye essentially behaves like a plus lens. The plus vergence of the eye can be excessive (resulting in myopia) or inadequate (resulting in hyperopia), both of which may be corrected by changing the total plus vergence to adequate levels. Of course, if the plus vergence is adequate, no lens correction is required.

Spherical lenses to correct refractive errors can be plus or minus, and are used to correct stigmatic refractive errors, such as myopia and hyperopia.

Myopic eyes have excessive plus vergence that needs to be decreased. This is accomplished by using minus lenses. Examples of lenses to correct myopia are:

> OD: –3.00 Sphere
> OS: –2.75 Sphere
> ("Sphere" is frequently shortened to SPH or Sph)

Hyperopic eyes have inadequate plus vergence that needs to be increased. This is accomplished by using plus lenses. Examples of lenses to correct hyperopia are:

OD: +3.00 Sphere
OS: +2.75 Sphere

Review Questions

1. All spherical lenses:
   a. have different powers along various meridians
   b. have the same power in all meridians
   c. only converge light
   d. only diverge light

2. A lens whose f is 50 cm and whose image forms in plus space is most likely:
   a. −2 D
   b. used to increase minus vergence
   c. used to increase plus vergence
   d. +5 D

3. A lens whose f is 0.5 m and whose image forms in minus space is most likely:
   a. −2 D
   b. used to decrease minus vergence
   c. used to increase plus vergence
   d. +5 D

4. Refractive error of a patient with excessive plus vergence may be corrected using:
   a. lenses that magnify images
   b. PL Sph
   c. lenses that reduce image sizes
   d. a +5 D lens

5. Refractive error of a patient with inadequate plus vergence may be corrected using:
   a. lenses that magnify images
   b. PL Sph
   c. lenses that reduce image sizes
   d. a −5 D lens

17

CYLINDRICAL LENSES

LEARNING OBJECTIVES

Upon completion of this chapter, the reader should be able to:

o   describe axis and power meridians.
o   describe use of cylindrical lenses to correct simple astigmatism.

KEY POINTS

o   Cylindrical lenses have two optical surfaces: a plane and a curved surface.
o   The plane surface has no curvature and no power; it is called the *cylinder axis*.
o   The curved surface has curvature and power; it is called the *power meridian*.
o   In cylindrical lenses, the cylinder axis and cylinder power are oriented at 90 degrees to each other.
o   Cylindrical lenses can be plus or minus, and will display characteristics of those lenses.
o   Plus or minus cylindrical lenses are used to correct simple astigmatic refractive errors such as simple myopic astigmatism (SMA) or simple hyperopic astigmatism (SHA).
o   Lens prescriptions for correcting simple astigmatic refractive errors will always have plano (PL) as one of the two sphere powers in transposed prescriptions.

CYLINDRICAL LENSES

Compared to spherical lenses, cylindrical (frequently shortened to "cylinder" or "cyl") lenses are somewhat more complex. Fortunately, many of the concepts described for spherical lenses may be modified for understanding cylindrical lenses.

Compared to spherical lenses, light rays in a cylindrical lens will converge or diverge only along one axis (meridian) because cylindrical lenses have two optical surfaces—a plane and a curved surface (Figure 17-1).

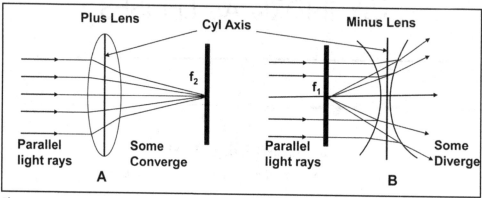

Figure 17-1. Astigmatic images by cylindrical lenses. Light rays in cylindrical lenses either converge or diverge along one axis (meridian), and images produced by cylindrical lenses form a line focus. The image produced by a plus cylindrical lens forms in the plus space of the lens (f_2), where some of the light rays converge (A). The image produced by a minus cylindrical lens appears to come from minus space of the lens (f_1), from where some of the light rays appear to diverge (B). Images in cylindrical lenses are produced parallel to the cylinder axis (Cyl Axis). In the examples shown, the cylinder axis is vertical and the power meridian is horizontal.

The plane surface has no curvature and no power. It is called the cylinder axis and is the location of the image of the curved surface, which is 90 degrees away. The curved surface has curvature and power; it is called the power meridian. Its image does not form a point focus (focal point), but rather a line focus (focal line) along the cylinder axis. Thus, in cylinder lenses, the cylinder axis and cylinder power meridian are oriented at 90 degrees to each other.

The image produced by a plus cylindrical lens forms a line focus in the plus space of the lens, where some of the light rays eventually converge (Figure 17-1A). The image produced by a minus cylindrical lens appears to come from a line focus in the minus space of the lens, from where some of the light rays appear to diverge (Figure 17-1B) (see Chapters 8 and 11).

Images formed by cylindrical lenses in this way are termed *astigmatic images* ("a" means "no" or "not").

Therefore, if a cylinder lens is oriented with its axis at 90, its full power is provided at axis 180. If the same lens is placed at some other axis, the full power will not be provided at 180, but at some other axis. Because of this, the cylinder axis is determined before cylinder power is measured during refractometry.

Example 1

At what axis will a cylinder lens of appropriate power be oriented to provide correction along axis 65?

Cylinder power required at axis: 65
Cylinder should be oriented 90 degrees away: 65 + 90 = 175

Thus, to provide power along axis 65, a cylinder lens of appropriate power must be oriented with its axis at 175.

Cylindrical lenses have two parameters—power and axis—and both are mutually at 90 degrees. Cylindrical lenses can be plus or minus, and will display characteristics of those lenses (eg, image movement, magnification, central and peripheral thickness, etc) (Chapter 8).

Concepts of speed of light, refractive index (RI), Snell's law, bending of light across an interface with different refractive indices, critical angle (i_c), total internal reflection (TIR), and prismatic nature of lenses described so far also apply to cylindrical lenses.

Focal length (f), diopters (D), vergence, and magnification may be calculated for cylindrical lenses using the formulae described in earlier chapters.

CORRECTION OF REFRACTIVE ERRORS (LENS PRESCRIPTIONS)

Cylindrical lenses can be plus or minus, and are used to correct astigmatic refractive errors in which only one meridian needs to be corrected (the other is plano [PL]). Such refractive errors are termed *simple astigmatism*, and two types may be identified depending on whether the meridian needing correction has excessive or inadequate plus power (Table 17-1).

Table 17-1			
Astigmatism	**Plus Power**	**Corrective Lens**	**Examples of Prescriptions**
Simple Myopic (SMA)	Appropriate along one axis; excessive 90 degrees away	Minus cylindrical	PL −1.00 x 180 A similar optical effect is obtained by using a plus cylindrical and a minus spherical lens: −1.00 +1.00 x 90
Simple Hyperopic (SHA)	Appropriate along one axis; inadequate 90 degrees away	Plus cylindrical	PL +1.00 x 90 A similar optical effect is obtained by using a minus cylindrical and a plus spherical lens: +1.00 −1.00 x 180

As shown in Table 17-1, SMA and SHA refractive errors may be measured using plus or minus cylinder refractors (Phoroptor). Lens prescriptions for correcting SMA and SHA may be readily identified by transposing a lens correction. One of the two spherical powers will always be PL.

Review Questions

1. If a +2.00 D cylindrical lens is placed with its axis at 77, at what axis will its power be fully effective?

    a. 77
    b. 167
    c. 90
    d. 180

2. If −1.00 D of cylindrical power is needed at axis 90, at what axis will you place the cylindrical lens?

    a. 77
    b. 167
    c. 90
    d. 180

3. What is the total cylindrical power if +1.00 D and −2.00 D cylindrical lenses are held with their axes parallel?

    a. −1 D
    b. +1 D
    c. −2 D
    d. +2 D

4. What is the total cylindrical power of a standard ±0.25 D Jackson Cross-Cylinder on a refractor (Phoroptor)?

    a. PL
    b. 0.25 D
    c. 0.5 D
    d. 0.75 D

5. What is the total cylindrical power if a +1.00 D cylindrical lens is held at axis 90, and a −1.00 D cylindrical lens is held at axis 180?

    a. PL
    b. +1 D
    c. +2 D
    d. +3 D

18

SPHEROCYLINDRICAL LENSES

LEARNING OBJECTIVES

Upon completion of this chapter, the reader should be able to:

o describe spherocylindrical lenses.

o describe the use of spherocylindrical lenses to correct compound astigmatism.

KEY POINTS

o Spherocylindrical lenses have two curved refractive surfaces.

o Spherocylindrical lenses can be either plus or minus, and are used to correct compound and mixed astigmatism.

o Lens prescriptions for correcting compound and mixed astigmatic refractive errors will never have plano (PL) as one of the two sphere powers in transposed prescriptions.

SPHEROCYLINDRICAL LENSES

As the name implies, a spherocylindrical lens is a combination of a spherical lens (see Chapter 16) and a cylindrical lens (see Chapter 17). Thus, spherocylindrical lenses have two meridians—one of maximum power and the other of minimum power.

Concepts of speed of light, refractive index (RI), Snell's Law, bending of light across an interface with two different refractive indices, critical angle (i_c), total internal reflection (TIR), and prismatic nature of lenses described so far also apply to spherocylindrical lenses.

Focal length (f), diopters (D), vergence, and magnification may be calculated for spherocylindrical lenses using the formulae described in earlier chapters.

TRANSPOSING SPHEROCYLINDRICAL LENS PRESCRIPTIONS

Spherocylindrical lens prescriptions include three parameters:

Sphere Power	Cylinder Power	X	Cylinder Axis

Since cylindrical lenses can be plus or minus, cylinder power can also be specified as plus or minus, and the lens prescription will be designated as plus cylinder or minus cylinder. Although there are exceptions, ophthalmologists (MDs and DOs) typically write lens prescriptions in plus cylinder form, whereas optometrists (ODs) typically write lens prescriptions in minus cylinder form.

	Sphere Power	Cylinder Power		Cylinder Axis	
+ cylinder form:	+3.00	+1.50	X	90	(commonly used by MDs and DOs)
– cylinder form:	+4.50	–1.50	X	180	(commonly used by ODs)

Lens prescriptions may be converted from plus cylinder to minus cylinder, and vice versa, by *transposing*. For example:

o   Plus cylinder to minus cylinder:

Plus cylinder:	+1.00	+2.00	X	90
	sphere	cylinder power		cylinder axis

Algebraically add the sphere and cylinder:	(+1) + (+2) = +3
New sphere power:	+3.00
Copy the full cylinder power:	2.00
Change the sign of the cylinder power:	–2.00
Change the axis by 90 (180 is the maximum):	(90 + 90 = 180)
The transposed Rx is:	

Minus cylinder:	+3.00	–2.00	X	180

o   Minus cylinder to plus cylinder:

Minus cylinder:	+2.00	–1.00	X	180
	sphere	cylinder power		cylinder axis

Algebraically add the sphere and cylinder:	(+2) + (–1) = +1
New sphere power:	+1.00
Copy the full cylinder power:	1.00
Change the sign of the cylinder power:	+1.00
Change the axis by 90 (180 is the maximum):	(180 – 90 = 90)
The transposed Rx is:	

Plus cylinder:	+1.00	+1.00	X	90

CORRECTION OF REFRACTIVE ERRORS (LENS PRESCRIPTIONS)

Spherocylindrical lenses are used to correct astigmatic refractive errors in which both meridians need to be corrected. Such refractive errors are termed *compound astigmatism* and *mixed astigmatism*. Two types of compound astigmatism may be identified depending on whether meridians have excessive or inadequate plus power (Table 18-1). Prescriptions in one form may be converted to the other form, as shown on the previous page.

Table 18-1

Astigmatism	Plus Power	Corrective Lens	Examples of Prescriptions
Compound Myopic (CMA)	Excessive along both axes	Minus spherical and minus cylindrical	–2.00 –1.00 x 180 A similar optical effect is obtained by using a minus spherical and a plus cylindrical lens: –3.00 +1.00 x 90
Compound Hyperopic (CHA)	Inadequate along both axes	Plus spherical and plus cylindrical	+2.00 +1.00 x 90 A similar optical effect is obtained by using a plus spherical and a minus cylindrical lens: +3.00 –1.00 x 180
Mixed (MA)	Excessive along one axis; inadequate 90 degrees away	Minus or plus spherical and cylindrical	+1.00 –3.00 x 180 or –2.00 +3.00 x 90

REVIEW QUESTIONS

1. The transposed form of +3.00 +1.50 x 90 is:
   a. +4.50 –1.50 x 90
   b. +3.75 –1.50 x 90
   c. +3.75 +1.50 x 180
   d. +4.50 –1.50 x 180

2. The transposed form of +4.00 +4.00 x 180 is:
   a. +8.00 –4.00 x 90
   b. +6.00 +4.00 x 90
   c. +6.00 +4.00 x 180
   d. +4.50 –1.50 x 180

3.   Spherocylindrical lenses have:
        a.   one plano surface
        b.   two refracting surfaces
        c.   two plano surfaces
        d.   one refracting surface

4.   Compound astigmatism may be corrected by:
        a.   spherocylindrical lenses
        b.   spherical lenses
        c.   cylinder lenses alone
        d.   plano lenses

5.   −2.00 +4.00 x 87 is an example of:
        a.   compound hyperopic astigmatism
        b.   compound myopic astigmatism
        c.   simple astigmatism
        d.   mixed astigmatism

19

OPTICAL CROSS

LEARNING OBJECTIVES

Upon completion of this chapter, the reader should be able to:

o   make an optical cross of a prescription, and vice versa.
o   obtain all relevant ophthalmic details from an optical cross.

KEY POINTS

o   Spherical, cylindrical, and spherocylindrical lens powers may be depicted in an optical cross.

o   An optical cross has two axes at 90 degrees to each other, representing two sphere powers that may be the same or different.

o   Optical crosses of spherical lenses have the same power in all axes.

o   Optical crosses of cylindrical lenses have no power along one meridian and all of the power along the other (ie, plano [PL] along one axis, and power along the other axis).

o   Optical crosses of spherocylindrical lenses are combinations of optical crosses of spherical lenses and minus or plus cylindrical lenses.

o   Optical crosses have clinical applications in lensometry, retinoscopy, refractometry, opticianry, and contact lenses.

o   The two sets of lensmeter lines correspond to the two axes in an optical cross.

o   Retinoscopy streaks correspond to the two axes in an optical cross.

o   Refractometry sphere, cylinder axis, cylinder power, and re-refined sphere powers may be considered to correspond to the two axes in an optical cross.

OPTICAL CROSS CONCEPT

Ophthalmic medical personnel (OMP), contact lens fitters, and opticians frequently depict lens prescriptions in an *optical cross* for the purpose of manipulations and calculations. Spherical, cylindrical, and spherocylindrical prescriptions may be depicted in this way.

The "cross" in an optical cross is made up of the two axes, mutually at 90 degrees to each other, representing the two sphere powers in a transposed lens prescription:

Lens prescription: **–2.00** +1.00 x 90*
Transposed: **–1.00** –1.00 x 180

Some practitioners prefer using three digits to denote cylinder axes. In this scheme, "90" will be noted as "090" and "5" as "005."

The two sphere powers, –2.00 and –1.00, may now be drawn on a power cross at the appropriate axis. The convention for axes (also termed *meridians*) is shown in Figure 19-1.

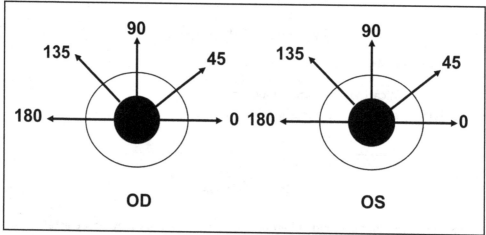

Figure 19–1. Convention for denoting axes in optical crosses, lens prescriptions, and ophthalmic discussions. Note that even though "0" is shown, it is actually never used, and is replaced by "180."

SPHERICAL LENS OPTICAL CROSS

Optical crosses of spherical lenses are the simplest. Since a spherical lens has the same power in all meridians, its optical cross will also have the same power along both axes (Figure 19-2).

Since the powers represented in the optical cross are the same in all meridians, any two axes may be used to depict the powers.

CYLINDRICAL LENS OPTICAL CROSS

Compared to optical crosses of spherical lenses, those of cylindrical lenses are somewhat more complicated. Since a cylindrical lens has no power along one meridian and all the power along the other, its optical cross will have plano (PL) along one axis, and power along the other axis (Figure 19-3).

Optical cross of a cylindrical lens may be used to derive a prescription in plus cylinder and minus cylinder form. Some practitioners prefer to use a degree symbol to denote the cylinder axis. In this scheme, "90" would be noted as "90°," and "180" as "180°."

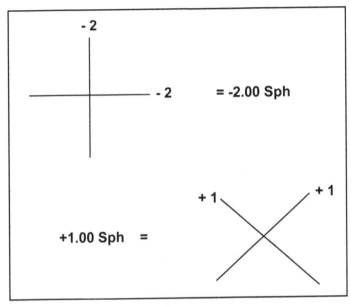

Figure 19–2. Optical cross of a spherical lens. Powers of both meridians are the same, and any pair of meridians may be used, such as 90 and 180 (top), or 45 and 135 (bottom).

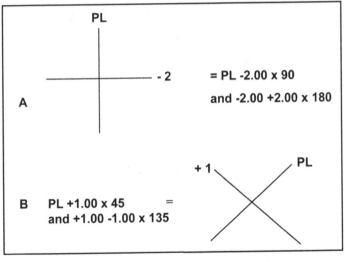

Figure 19–3. Optical cross of a cylindrical lens. One meridian always has PL power and denotes the cylinder axis. The other meridian is the power meridian. The lens prescription may be derived from the optical cross (top), and a lens prescription may be depicted by an optical cross (bottom).

SPHEROCYLINDRICAL LENS OPTICAL CROSS

As the name indicates, a spherocylindrical lens is a combination of a spherical lens and a cylindrical lens. The optical cross of a spherocylindrical lens is a combination of the optical crosses of a spherical lens and a minus or plus cylindrical lens (Figure 19-4).

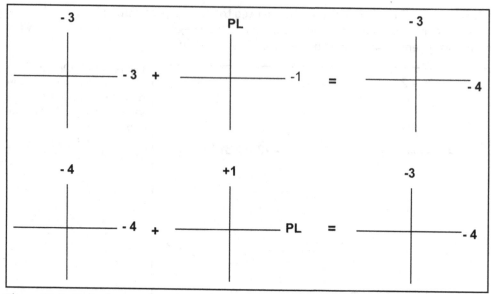

Figure 19-4. Optical cross of a spherocylindrical lens is a combination of the optical cross of a spherical lens and an optical cross of a minus cylindrical lens (top) or a plus cylindrical lens (bottom).

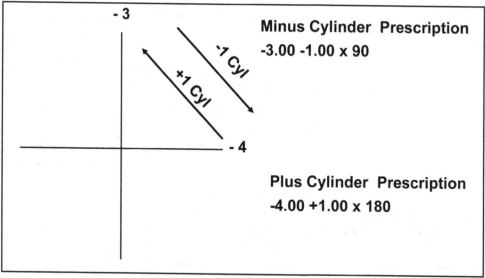

Figure 19-5. Plus and minus cylindrical lens prescriptions derived from an optical cross. A –1 D cylindrical lens at axis 90 in combination with a –3 D spherical lens results in a minus cylinder prescription (top); whereas a +1 D cylindrical lens at axis 180 in combination with a –4 D spherical lens results in a plus cylinder prescription (bottom).

Plus and minus cylinder prescriptions may be derived from an optical cross (Figure 19-5). Once an optical cross has been drawn showing spherical lenses at the two axes, a cylindrical lens can be added to one axis so that its power, in combination with the spherical lens at that axis, yields the total power at the second axis. Similarly, a cylindrical lens can be added to the second axis so that its power, in combination with the spherical lens at that axis, yields the total power at the first axis. The two cylindrical lenses should be of the same power but with opposite signs.

A minus cylinder prescription results from combining a minus cylindrical lens at an axis with a spherical lens (Figure 19-5, top), whereas a plus cylinder prescription results from combining a plus cylindrical lens at an axis with a spherical lens (Figure 19-5, bottom).

Example 1

Draw an optical cross showing all of the optical details of the following lens prescription (Figure 19-6).

$$+2.75 \ +1.50 \ x \ 80$$

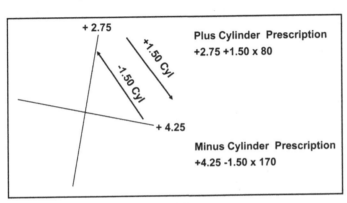

Plus Cylinder Prescription
+2.75 +1.50 x 80

Minus Cylinder Prescription
+4.25 -1.50 x 170

Figure 19-6. Optical cross showing optical details of a plus cylinder lens prescription, +2.75 +1.50 x 80 (top), and a minus cylinder prescription, +4.25 −1.50 x 170 (bottom).

Example 2

Derive plus cylinder and minus cylinder lens prescriptions from the following optical cross (Figure 19-7).

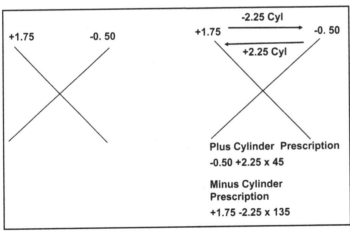

Plus Cylinder Prescription
-0.50 +2.25 x 45

Minus Cylinder Prescription
+1.75 -2.25 x 135

Figure 19-7. Optical cross (left) showing plus and minus cylinder prescriptions and other optical details derived from it (right).

CLINICAL APPLICATIONS

Optical crosses are a useful tool with clinical applications in lensometry, retinoscopy, and refractometry.

LENSOMETRY

Reading glasses and rigid gas-permeable (RGP) contact lens powers in a lensmeter is very similar to drawing an optical cross. The two sets of lensmeter lines (thin and closer set, and thick and farther apart set) are like the two axes in an optical cross, and may be used to determine various optical and refractive parameters of lenses (Table 19-1).

Table 19-1		
Lens	**Lensmeter**	**Optical Cross**
Spherical lens	Thin and thick lines in focus simultaneously.	Same power in both axes
Cylindrical lens	Two sets of lines do not focus simultaneously. In transposed prescriptions one reading will always be plano; the other has power; OR sphere and cylinder powers are similar but of opposite sign.	One axis is plane; the other has power
Spherocylindrical lens	Two sets of lines do not focus simultaneously. Both readings have power; cylinder power may be less than, the same as, or greater than the sphere power.	Both axes have power

A comparison of characteristics of spherocylindrical lenses, as depicted in optical crosses and seen in *lensometry*, is shown in Figure 19-8.

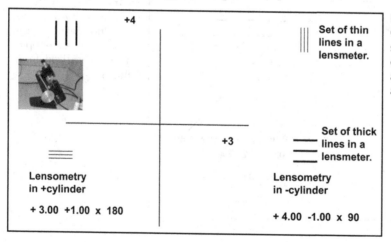

Figure 19-8. Comparison of spherocylindrical characteristics in an optical cross and lensometry.

Retinoscopy

Retinoscopy is an objective method to measure refractive errors in patients who are unable to respond subjectively (eg, infants, preschool toddlers, and adults unable to communicate).

The light from the retinoscope is termed the *intercept*, whereas the light reflected from the fundus and observed through the pupil is termed the *streak*. This terminology will be followed ahead. Standard textbooks (see References) should be consulted for additional details of retinoscopy.

Retinoscopy is particularly useful in a pediatric ophthalmic clinic where a rapid measurement of refractive errors is necessary. As described in Chapter 9, the collar of a streak retinoscope may be moved vertically in order to provide positive vergence (plus power) to estimate the degree of hyperopia along any meridian that shows with motion of the streak.[1] This setting of the retinoscope is termed the *concave-mirror effect*, and is achieved by moving the collar vertically upwards in a Welch-Allyn retinoscope and vertically downwards in a Copeland retinoscope. The required amount of plus power is indicated when the streak is the sharpest. The maximum amount of plus power that can be provided by a streak retinoscope is +5 D when the collar is moved halfway, while moving the collar ¼ way provides +2.50 D. The direction of movement of the intercept (NOT its orientation) indicates the optical axis:

o   Intercept oriented vertically but moved horizontally
   =   vertical streak   =   indicates axis 180

o   Intercept oriented horizontally but moved vertically
   =   horizontal streak   =   indicates axis 90

o   Intercept oriented obliquely (eg, axis 135) but moved along axis 45
   =   oblique streak   =   indicates axis 45

o   Intercept oriented obliquely (eg, axis 45) but moved along axis 135
   =   oblique streak   =   indicates axis 135

Once the two axes have been neutralized, we know the two variables necessary to create an optical cross (axis and power), and may obtain lens prescriptions in plus and minus cylinders (Figure 19-9).

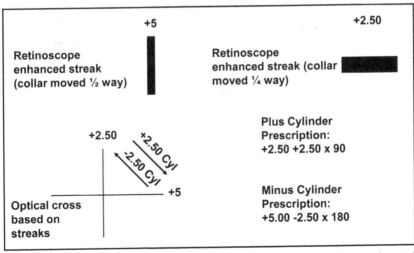

Figure 19-9. Plus and minus cylinder lens prescriptions obtained from enhanced streaks in objective retinoscopy.

Refractometry

Refractometry is a subjective method to measure refractive errors in patients who are able to respond (eg, older children and adults able to communicate).

Standard textbooks (see Reference) should be consulted for details of refractometry.

A standard refractor (Phoroptor) or trial lenses are used to measure refractive errors using the following six steps:

1. Refine sphere power
2. Refine cylinder axis
3. Refine cylinder power   } Can be depicted in an optical cross
4. Re-refine sphere
5. Red-green (duochrome) test
6. Balancing (if necessary)

A refractive error measurement obtained by refractometry may be depicted in an optical cross (Figure 19-10).

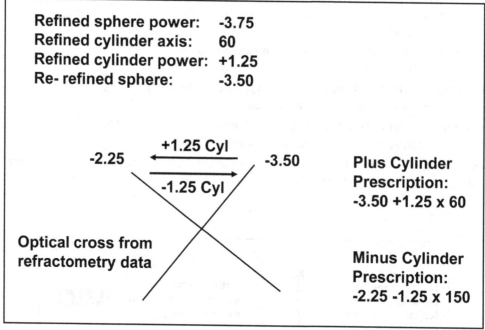

Refined sphere power: -3.75
Refined cylinder axis: 60
Refined cylinder power: +1.25
Re- refined sphere: -3.50

-2.25   +1.25 Cyl   -3.50
                -1.25 Cyl

Plus Cylinder Prescription:
-3.50 +1.25 x 60

Optical cross from refractometry data

Minus Cylinder Prescription:
-2.25 -1.25 x 150

Figure 19-10. Optical cross and plus and minus cylinder lens prescriptions obtained from subjective refractometry.

Reference

1. Corboy JM. *The Retinoscopy Book: An Introductory Manual for Eye Care Professionals*. Thorofare, NJ: SLACK Incorporated; 2003.

Review Questions

1.   The following optical cross represents a:

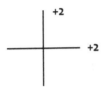

      a.   cylindrical lens with axis at 90
      b.   spherical lens
      c.   cylindrical lens with axis at 180
      d.   spherocylindrical lens

2.   The following optical cross represents a:

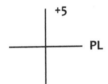

      a.   cylindrical lens with axis at 90
      b.   spherical lens
      c.   cylindrical lens with axis at 180
      d.   spherocylindrical lens

3.   The following optical cross represents a:

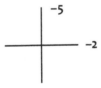

      a.   cylindrical lens with axis at 90
      b.   spherical lens
      c.   cylindrical lens with axis at 180
      d.   spherocylindrical lens

4. What is the prescription of a spherocylindrical lens depicted by the following optical crosses?

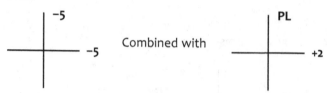

   a.   +5.00 –2.00 x 90
   b.   –3.00 –2.00 x 180
   c.   –5.00 +2.00 x 180
   d.   +3.00 +2.00 x 90

5. The optical cross depicting the prescription –1.00 +3.00 x 90 is:

   a.

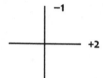

   b.

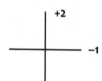

   c.

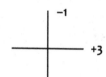

   d.

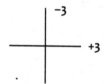

20

CONOID OF STURM

LEARNING Objectives

Upon completion of this chapter, the reader should be able to:

o   describe formation of images in the Conoid of Sturm.
o   describe the Circle of Least Confusion and spherical equivalent.
o   calculate the spherical equivalent.

KEY POINTS

o   In spherocylindrical lenses, vertical and horizontal light rays converge to form a cone.
o   Separate images are produced along the two axes depending on their powers.
o   The interval between the two images is called the Conoid of Sturm.
o   The midpoint of the Conoid of Sturm is termed the *Circle of Least Confusion*.
o   The dioptric equivalent to the Circle of Least Confusion is the spherical equivalent.
o   In spherocylindrical lens prescriptions, the spherical equivalent is calculated by algebraically adding half the cylinder power to the sphere power.

IMAGES OF SPHEROCYLINDRICAL LENSES

As described in Chapter 18, a spherocylindrical lens produces two line foci oriented at 90 degrees to each other. Thus, the two images are also positioned mutually at 90 degrees to each other and at the focal length of the two axes. For example, in a spherocylindrical lens with axes with powers of +2 D and +4 D, the image of the +2 D axis will form at 50 cm from the lens, while the image of the +4 D axis will form at 25 cm from the lens (Figure 20-1). In addition, light rays traveling parallel to one axis produce an image parallel to the other axis, and vice versa. Vertical and horizontal light rays form cones in which light rays converge to produce images.

Thus,

Light parallel to axis 90	=	image produced parallel to axis 180
Light parallel to axis 180	=	image produced parallel to axis 90
Light parallel to axis 45	=	image produced parallel to axis 135
Light parallel to axis 135	=	image produced parallel to axis 45

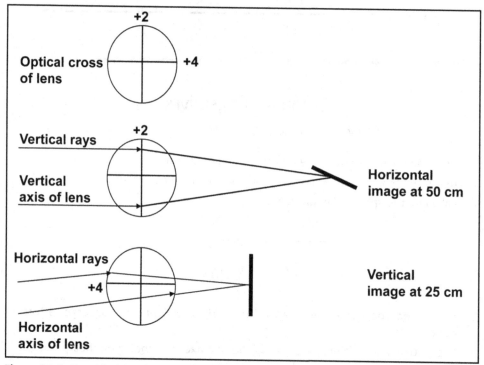

Figure 20-1. Conoid of Sturm in a spherocylindrical lens. In the optical cross (top), the vertical light rays form a cone and a horizontal image (middle), whereas the horizontal light rays form a cone and a vertical image (bottom).

CONOID OF STURM

The interval between the two images produced by a spherocylindrical lens is called the *Conoid of Sturm* because light rays connecting the two line foci form a cone. The Conoid of Sturm is also termed the Interval of Sturm or Sturm's Conoid.

Cross sections of the Conoid along its length are ellipses. The midpoint of this interval is termed the *Circle of Least Confusion*. The Circle of Least Confusion represents the position of the least blurry image within the Conoid, and its cross section is circular (hence "circle" of least confusion) (Figure 20-2).

The dioptric equivalent to the Circle of Least Confusion is termed the *spherical equivalent*, and it represents the power of a spherical lens used in place of the spherocylindrical lens. In spherocylindrical lens prescriptions, the spherical equivalent may be calculated by algebraically adding half of the cylinder power to the sphere power.

The concepts of Conoid of Sturm and the Circle of Least Confusion have direct applications in considering regular astigmatism, and readers are encouraged to see Chapter 24 for those details.

The concept of spherical equivalent has clinical applications in refractometry and is used for determining the power of a non-toric soft contact lens (SCL) from a prescription that includes minor amounts of astigmatism (see ahead).

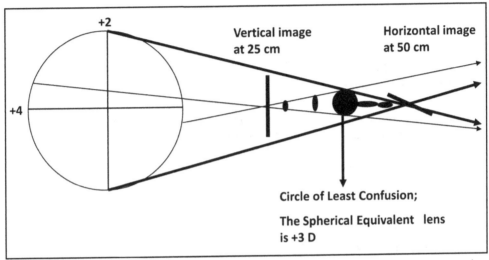

Figure 20-2. Conoid of Sturm in a spherocylindrical lens. Space between the two images has elliptical images. Midway between the two images is a circular area termed the Circle of Least Confusion, and it represents the "spherical equivalent," or the dioptric power, of a spherical lens that will produce the best image in place of the spherocylindrical lens.

CALCULATING SPHERICAL EQUIVALENT

The spherical equivalent, located midway in the Conoid of Sturm, is the dioptric value of the Circle of Least Confusion. The spherical equivalent in any spherocylindrical lens prescription may be calculated by algebraically adding half of the cylinder power to the sphere power:

EXAMPLE 1

Lens prescription:	+3.00 +0.50 x 90
Half cylinder power:	$\frac{0.50}{2}$
Half cylinder power:	+0.25
Sphere power:	+3.00
Spherical equivalent:	(Sphere power) + (Half cylinder power)
Spherical equivalent:	(+3) + (+0.25)
Spherical equivalent:	+3 + 0.25
Spherical equivalent:	+3.25

Example 2

Lens prescription:	+3.50 −0.50 x 150
Half cylinder power:	$\frac{-0.50}{2}$
Half cylinder power:	−0.25
Sphere power:	+3.50
Spherical equivalent:	(Sphere power) + (Half cylinder power)
Spherical equivalent:	(+3.50) + (−0.25)
Spherical equivalent:	+3.50 − 0.25
Spherical equivalent:	+3.25

Example 3

Lens prescription:	−2.75 −0.50 x 170
Half cylinder power:	$\frac{-0.50}{2}$
Half cylinder power:	−0.25
Sphere power:	−2.75
Spherical equivalent:	(Sphere power) + (Half cylinder power)
Spherical equivalent:	(−2.75) + (−0.25)
Spherical equivalent:	−2.75 − 0.25
Spherical equivalent:	−3.00

Example 4

Lens prescription:	−3.25 +0.50 x 170
Half cylinder power:	$\frac{0.50}{2}$
Half cylinder power:	+0.25
Sphere power:	−3.25
Spherical equivalent:	(Sphere power) + (Half cylinder power)
Spherical equivalent:	(−3.25) + (+0.25)
Spherical equivalent:	−3.25 + 0.25
Spherical equivalent:	−3.00

CLINICAL APPLICATIONS

The concepts of the Circle of Least Confusion and spherical equivalent, which are based on the Conoid of Sturm, have important clinical applications in refractometry and non-toric SCL.

Spherical Equivalent and Refractometry

The concepts of the Circle of Least Confusion and spherical equivalent are used during measurements of compound and mixed astigmatic refractive errors by *manifest refractometry* (MR) or *cycloplegic refractometry* (CR).

When refining a spherocylindrical lens prescription for compound myopic astigmatism (eg, −2.00 +0.50 x 85) from retinoscopy or the current spectacle lenses, the goal of refractometry is to move the two line foci toward the Circle of Least Confusion, thus collapsing the Conoid of Sturm on the fovea to produce the sharpest image possible. This goal may be achieved using a plus or minus cylinder refractor (Phoroptor) (Figure 20-3).

Similar manipulations may be accomplished for compound hyperopic astigmatism and mixed astigmatism (Figures 20-4 and 20-5).

Spherical Equivalent and Soft Contact Lenses

For minor amounts of astigmatism, spherical SCL may be considered instead of toric SCL because spherical lenses may provide acceptably good visual acuity, and their fitting does not have the potential for as many complications as toric SCL.

Readers are encouraged to consult standard references for reviewing guidelines established for considering spherical SCL instead of toric SCL.

Example 5

Lens prescription:	−2.50 +0.50 X 50
Convert to minus cylinder:	−2.00 −0.50 X 140
Spherical equivalent:	(Sphere power) + (Half cylinder power)
Spherical equivalent:	$(-2.00) + (\frac{-0.50}{2})$
Spherical equivalent:	$(-2.00) + (-0.25)$
Spherical equivalent:	−2.00 − 0.25
Spherical soft lens power:	−2.25

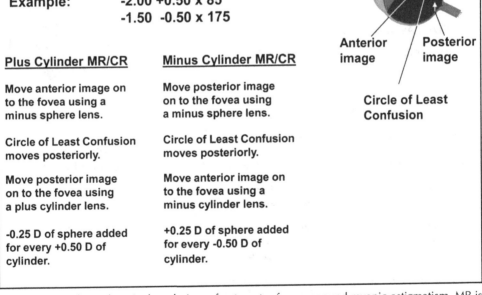

Compound Myopic Astigmatism

Example: -2.00 +0.50 x 85
-1.50 -0.50 x 175

Anterior image   Posterior image

Circle of Least Confusion

Plus Cylinder MR/CR	**Minus Cylinder MR/CR**
Move anterior image on to the fovea using a minus sphere lens.	Move posterior image on to the fovea using a minus sphere lens.
Circle of Least Confusion moves posteriorly.	Circle of Least Confusion moves posteriorly.
Move posterior image on to the fovea using a plus cylinder lens.	Move anterior image on to the fovea using a minus cylinder lens.
-0.25 D of sphere added for every +0.50 D of cylinder.	+0.25 D of sphere added for every -0.50 D of cylinder.

Figure 20-3. Spherical equivalent during refractometry for compound myopic astigmatism. MR is manifest refractometry; CR is cycloplegic refractometry.

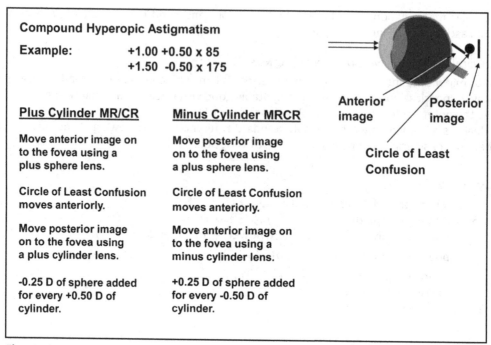

Compound Hyperopic Astigmatism

Example: +1.00 +0.50 x 85
                  +1.50 -0.50 x 175

Anterior   Posterior
image   image

Circle of Least
Confusion

<u>Plus Cylinder MR/CR</u>

Move anterior image on
to the fovea using a
plus sphere lens.

Circle of Least Confusion
moves anteriorly.

Move posterior image
on to the fovea using
a plus cylinder lens.

-0.25 D of sphere added
for every +0.50 D of
cylinder.

<u>Minus Cylinder MRCR</u>

Move posterior image
on to the fovea using
a plus sphere lens.

Circle of Least Confusion
moves anteriorly.

Move anterior image on
to the fovea using a
minus cylinder lens.

+0.25 D of sphere added
for every -0.50 D of
cylinder.

Figure 20-4. Spherical equivalent during refractometry for compound hyperopic astigmatism. MR is manifest refractometry; CR is cycloplegic refractometry.

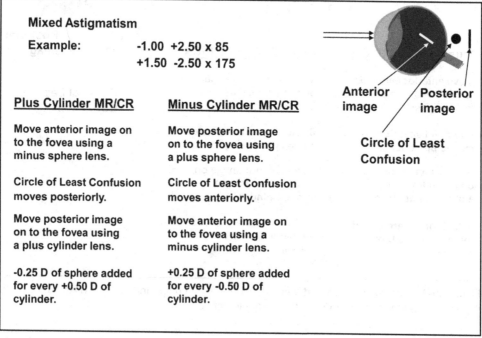

Mixed Astigmatism

Example: -1.00 +2.50 x 85
                  +1.50 -2.50 x 175

Anterior   Posterior
image   image

Circle of Least
Confusion

<u>Plus Cylinder MR/CR</u>

Move anterior image on
to the fovea using a
minus sphere lens.

Circle of Least Confusion
moves posteriorly.

Move posterior image
on to the fovea using
a plus cylinder lens.

-0.25 D of sphere added
for every +0.50 D of
cylinder.

<u>Minus Cylinder MR/CR</u>

Move posterior image
on to the fovea using
a plus sphere lens.

Circle of Least Confusion
moves anteriorly.

Move anterior image on
to the fovea using a
minus cylinder lens.

+0.25 D of sphere added
for every -0.50 D of
cylinder.

Figure 20-5. Spherical equivalent during refractometry for mixed astigmatism. MR is manifest refractometry; CR is cycloplegic refractometry.

Example 6

Lens prescription:	+3.00 +1.00 x 75
Convert to minus cylinder:	+4.00 −1.00 x 165
Spherical equivalent:	(Sphere power) + (Half cylinder power)
Spherical equivalent:	$(+4.00) + (\frac{-1.00}{2})$
Spherical equivalent:	(+4.00) + (−0.50)
Spherical equivalent:	+4.00 − 0.50
Spherical soft lens power:	+3.50

Review Questions

1. What is the spherical equivalent in the lens prescription +4.00 −2.00 x 90?
    - a. −2.00
    - b. +3.00
    - c. +2.00
    - d. −3.00

2. What is the spherical equivalent in the lens prescription +4.00 +1.00 x 90?
    - a. −4.00
    - b. +5.00
    - c. +4.50
    - d. +1.00

3. What is the spherical equivalent in the lens prescription PL +0.50 x 75?
    - a. −0.25
    - b. −0.50
    - c. +0.25
    - d. +0.50

4. A spherical soft lens for the spherocylindrical lens prescription −1.75 −0.50 x 55 is:
    - a. −2.25
    - b. −1.75
    - c. −2.75
    - d. −2.00

5. A spherical soft lens for the spherocylindrical lens prescription −2.50 +0.50 x 100 is:
    - a. −2.25
    - b. −1.75
    - c. −2.00
    - d. −2.50

21

OPTICAL SYSTEM OF THE HUMAN EYE

LEARNING Objectives

Upon completion of this chapter, the reader should be able to:

o   describe optics of the human eye.
o   describe the human eye as a lens and refracting system.

KEY POINTS

o   The human eye has five optical media for refraction: tears, cornea, aqueous, crystalline lens, and vitreous.
o   The total refraction at all the interfaces establishes presence of emmetropia or ametropia.
o   Optical media of the eye have specific refractive indices (RI) (air = 1.000): water (1.300); tears (1.336); aqueous (1.336); cornea (1.376); lens (1.386); and vitreous (1.336).
o   Simplified values of the schematic reduced (or reduced) eye may be used for calculations.

OPTICAL MEDIA OF THE EYE

Previous chapters described the basics of light and optics (refractive index [RI], Snell's law, refraction, and reflection) and applied those concepts to lenses, prisms, and mirrors.

Now, we move on and apply RI, Snell's law, and refraction to the human eye to investigate how light passes into the eye in order to produce a sharp image.

The human eye has five *optical media*, and light is refracted at the interfaces between those media (Table 21-1).

Table 21-1	
Optical Medium	**Interface for Light Refraction**
Tears	Air-tears
Cornea	Tears-anterior cornea
Aqueous	Posterior cornea-aqueous
Crystalline Lens	Aqueous-anterior lens
Vitreous	Posterior lens-vitreous

Refraction of light occurs at each of the interfaces, and the total of these refractions establishes the refractive status of the eye—emmetropia or ametropia.

REFRACTIVE INDICES OF OPTICAL MEDIA IN THE EYE

Table 21-2 lists the RI of optical media involved in light refraction by the eye and formation of images on the fovea.[1]

Table 21-2	
Optical Medium	**Refractive Index**
Air	1.000
Tears	1.336
Cornea	1.376
Aqueous	1.336
Crystalline Lens	1.386
Vitreous	1.336

Readers are encouraged to remember the RI of various optical media in order to properly complete calculations that might be required in clinical work. In the next chapter, we will apply these values to calculate the refracting powers of curved surfaces.

SCHEMATIC REDUCED EYE

Any system consisting of many lenses can be simplified to a few critical items in order to facilitate calculations. The concept of simplifying the complexities of the human eye was described by many authors, and the most widely used is the one described by Gullstrand.[1]

The *schematic reduced eye* (or reduced eye) simplifies the refraction of all of the ocular media, and interfaces into a single refracting entity. In Gullstrand's reduced eye, the axial length is assumed to be 24.4 mm.

The reduced eye may be used for optical calculations by using its simplified values.

Reference

1. Thall EH, Miller KM, Rosenthal P, Schechter RJ, Steinert RF, Beardsley TL. *Basic and Clinical Science Course, Section 3: Optics, Refraction, and Contact Lenses*. San Francisco, CA: American Academy of Ophthalmology; 2000.

Review Questions

1. The total number of optical media in the eye is:
   - a. 2
   - b. 5
   - c. 4
   - d. 3

2. Refractive interfaces in the eye include:
   - a. posterior cornea-anterior cornea; posterior lens-vitreous; tears-aqueous
   - b. air-tears; anterior cornea-posterior cornea
   - c. tears-vitreous; anterior cornea-air; aqueous-vitreous; air-vitreous
   - d. air-tears; tears-anterior cornea; posterior cornea-aqueous

3. Appropriate amount of refraction at all the interfaces establishes:
   - a. emmetropia
   - b. simple astigmatism
   - c. ametropia
   - d. compound astigmatism

4. Simplifying the complexities of refraction in the eye results in a/an:
   - a. emmetropic eye
   - b. refractive eye
   - c. schematic reduced eye
   - d. ametropic eye

5. The axial length assigned by Gullstrand is:
   - a. 24 cm
   - b. 24 m
   - c. 2.44 cm
   - d. 2.44 mm

22

REFRACTING POWER OF A CURVED SURFACE

LEARNING Objectives

Upon completion of this chapter, the reader should be able to:

o describe the effect of radius of curvature on refraction.
o calculate the power of a curved surface.
o calculate the power of ocular surfaces.

Key Points

o Tears, cornea, aqueous, lens, and vitreous have curved surfaces, which introduces the final variable in refraction in the eye: radius of curvature (r).

o The refracting power of a curved surface is a function of its r and the refractive index (RI) of the two media across the curved surface.

o If the r decreases, the refractive power will increase. If the r increases, the refractive power will decrease.

o The air-tear-anterior cornea surfaces together provide positive vergence (plus power).

o The posterior cornea-aqueous surface provides negative vergence (minus power).

o Both surfaces of the crystalline lens provide positive vergence (plus power).

o The air-anterior spectacle lens surface provides positive vergence (plus power).

o The posterior spectacle lens-air surface provides negative vergence (minus power).

o The air-tear surface provides the greatest plus power to incoming light rays.

KEY POINTS (CONTINUED)

o   Blurry vision due to dry eyes is due to loss of the plus power of the air-tear sur-
    face.

o   Patients with refractive corrections of ≥4 D often complain of discomfort with a
    base curve different from their habitual spectacle lenses.

o   Diabetes mellitus can produce 3 to 4 D of hyperopic and myopic shifts due to varia-
    tions in blood glucose.

o   Refractive surgery for eliminating myopia or hyperopia changes corneal curva-
    tures.

o   Corneal curvatures measured in keratometry may be converted from diopters (D)
    to mm of r.

o   The base curve of a contact lens is the central posterior curve, which has a specific r.

THE FINAL VARIABLE

So far, we have been dealing with variables such as refractive index (RI) and Snell's law,
associated with refraction at plane (uncurved) surfaces. These variables were also applied to
refraction in the eye in order to establish its refractive status (emmetropia and ametropia).

The final piece of this puzzle, and where our optical "journey" will begin its end, is to
apply all of these concepts to refraction by the tears, cornea, aqueous, crystalline lens, and
vitreous. Since all of these surfaces are curved, this chapter will introduce the final variable in
refraction in the eye: radius of curvature (r) and refractive power of curved surfaces.

Although the term radius of curvature sounds complicated, ophthalmic medical personnel
(OMP) deal with it every day because it is also known as the *base curve* of glasses and contact
lenses and is the basis of the ophthalmometer (Keratometer). The "8.4" or "8.6" base curve
OMP mention each day in the clinic when fitting soft contact lenses (SCL) refers to the r in
mm of the contact lens.

REFRACTING POWER OF A CURVED SURFACE

While Snell's law applies to all light rays entering the eye, the r of the cornea (and, therefore, tear film) adds the final variable to light refraction. Similarly, the power of lenses varies
depending on their r.

The refracting power of a curved surface is a function of:

o   the r of the curved surface

o   the RI of the two media on both sides of the curved surface

These factors can be expressed mathematically by:

$$P_{(D)} = \frac{(n_2 - n_1)}{r_{(m)}}$$

Where:

P = refractive power in diopters (D)

n_1 = RI of the medium from which light is coming (first medium)

n_2 = RI of the medium into which light is going (second medium)

r = radius of curvature (in m) of refractive surface

Since the r of the cornea and lenses is typically specified in mm, the formula can be rearranged to consider r in mm for ease of calculations. Since there are 1000 mm in 1 m, the numerator and denominator are multiplied by 1000, and the formula becomes:

$$P_{(D)} = \frac{1000\,(n_2 - n_1)}{1000\,r_{(m)}} = \frac{1000\,(n_2 - n_1)}{r_{(mm)}}$$

Where:

P = refractive power in D

n_1 = RI of the medium from which light is coming (first medium)

n_2 = RI of the medium into which light is going (second medium)

r = radius of curvature (in mm) of refractive surface

Therefore, if the r decreases, the refractive power will increase. If the r increases, the refractive power will decrease. Vergence and power changes as described occur whether light enters or exits the eye.

REFRACTION BY THE CURVED SURFACES OF THE AIR-TEAR-CORNEA COMPLEX

In addition to the power changes due to variations in r of the curved surface, the surface will also provide vergence changes. Whether vergence is positive (plus power) or negative (minus power) depends on the curvature of the surface between two refracting media[1]:

o   If the refractive surface with the greater RI medium is convex, vergence will be positive (plus power).

o   If the refractive surface with the greater RI medium is concave, vergence will be negative (minus power).

Using the scheme described above, it will be seen that the curved surfaces of the air-tear-anterior cornea complex together provide positive vergence (plus power), whereas the posterior cornea-aqueous curved surface provides negative vergence (minus power) (Figure 22-1). Vergence and powers as described occur whether light enters or exits the eye.

REFRACTION BY THE CURVED SURFACES OF THE CRYSTALLINE LENS

Both surfaces of the crystalline lens are convex, and the RI of the lens is greater than aqueous and vitreous. Based on the scheme described above, both surfaces of the crystalline lens provide positive vergence (plus power) (Figure 22-2). Vergence and powers as described occur whether light enters or exits the eye.

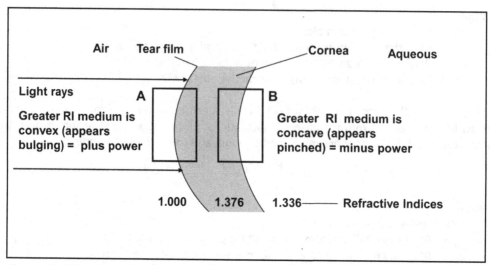

Figure 22-1. Vergence changes to light rays by the air-tears-cornea-aqueous combination. If the medium with the greater refractive index (RI) is convex, it provides positive vergence (plus power) (A); whereas if the medium with greater RI is concave, it provides negative vergence (minus power) (B). RI shown are for air (1.000), cornea (1.376), and aqueous (1.336). RI of tears is the same as aqueous. Refractive indices from Thall et al.[2]

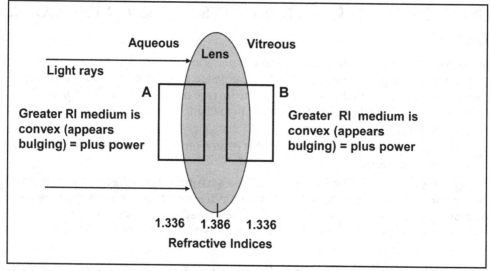

Figure 22-2. Vergence changes to light rays by the crystalline lens. The crystalline lens has the greater refractive index (RI), and is convex on both sides (A and B). Therefore, both surfaces provide positive vergence (plus power). Refractive indices from Thall et al.[2]

REFRACTION BY SPECTACLE LENSES

In terms of vergence (positive and negative) and power (plus and minus), a spectacle lens is optically similar to the tears-cornea-aqueous combination. Both surfaces of a spectacle lens are curved. The air-anterior spectacle lens surface is convex and provides positive vergence (plus power), whereas negative vergence (minus power) is provided by the posterior spectacle lens-air surface, which is concave (Figure 22-3). Vergence and powers as described occur when light passes through a spectacle lens in both directions.

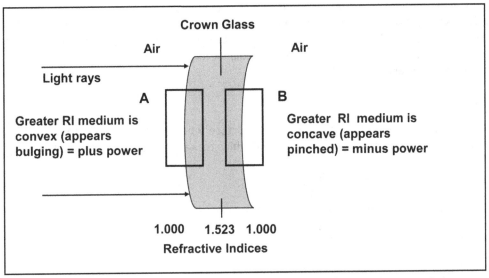

Figure 22-3. Vergence changes to light rays by spectacle lenses. The anterior spectacle lens surface is convex and its refractive index (RI) is greater than air (A); it therefore provides positive vergence (plus power). The posterior spectacle lens surface is concave and its RI is greater than air (B); it provides negative vergence (minus power). Refractive indices from Thall et al.[2]

SUMMARY OF ALL REFRACTIVE SURFACES INVOLVED WITH THE EYE

Vergence and power changes provided by the five curved surfaces of the eye are summarized in Table 22-1. Vergence and powers as described occur whether light enters or exits the eye or passes through a spectacle lens in either direction.

Table 22-1		
Optical Medium	**Surface for Light Refraction**	**Vergence (Power)**
Tears	Air-tears	Positive (plus)
Cornea	Tears-anterior cornea	Positive (plus)
Aqueous	Posterior cornea-aqueous	Negative (minus)
Crystalline Lens	Aqueous-anterior lens	Positive (plus)
Vitreous	Posterior lens-vitreous	Positive (plus)
Spectacle Lens	Air-anterior spectacle lens	Positive (plus)
Spectacle Lens	Posterior spectacle lens-air	Negative (minus)

CALCULATING REFRACTIVE POWERS OF CURVED SURFACES IN THE EYE

Refraction of light to produce retinal images occurs at the five curved surfaces described above, and the vergence and power (in D) of each surface contributes to the total refraction of light in the eye (Table 22-2). These values are obtained using the formula described above with standard values for RI and r of various media.[2,3] Vergence and powers as described occur whether light enters or exits the eye.

EXAMPLE 1

What is the power of the air-tear curved surface when light rays enter the eye? [RI: air (1.000), tears (1.336); r of the anterior cornea, which makes the tear film curved: 7.7 mm.[2]]

$$n_1 = \text{air}$$
$$n_1 = 1.000$$
$$n_2 = \text{tears}$$
$$n_2 = 1.336$$
$$r = 7.7 \text{ mm}$$

$$P_{(D)} = \frac{1000 \, (n_2 - n_1)}{r(mm)}$$
$$P_{(D)} = \frac{1000 \, (1.336 - 1.000)}{7.7}$$
$$P_{(D)} = \frac{1000 \, (0.336)}{7.7}$$
$$P_{(D)} = \frac{336}{7.7}$$
$$P_{(D)} = +43.6 \text{ D}$$

EXAMPLE 2

What is the power of the tear-anterior cornea curved surface when light rays enter the eye? [RI: tears (1.336), cornea (1.376); r of the anterior cornea: 7.7 mm.[2]]

$$n_1 = \text{tears}$$
$$n_1 = 1.336$$
$$n_2 = \text{cornea}$$
$$n_2 = 1.376$$
$$r = 7.7 \text{ mm}$$

$$P_{(D)} = \frac{1000 \, (n_2 - n_1)}{r(mm)}$$
$$P_{(D)} = \frac{1000 \, (1.376 - 1.336)}{7.7}$$
$$P_{(D)} = \frac{1000 \, (0.040)}{7.7}$$
$$P_{(D)} = \frac{40}{7.7}$$
$$P_{(D)} = +5.2 \text{ D}$$

Example 3

What is the power of the posterior cornea-aqueous curved surface when light rays enter the eye? [RI: cornea (1.376), aqueous (1.336); r of the posterior cornea: 6.8 mm.[2]]

$$n_1 = \text{cornea}$$
$$n_1 = 1.376$$
$$n_2 = \text{aqueous}$$
$$n_2 = 1.336$$
$$r = 6.8 \text{ mm}$$

$$P_{(D)} = \frac{1000\,(n_2 - n_1)}{r(mm)}$$

$$P_{(D)} = \frac{1000\,(1.336 - 1.376)}{6.8}$$

$$P_{(D)} = \frac{1000\,(-0.040)}{6.8}$$

$$P_{(D)} = \frac{-40}{6.8}$$

$$P_{(D)} = -5.8 \text{ D}$$

Table 22-2		
Media	**Surface for Light Refraction**	**Vergence (Power; D)**
Tears	Air-tears	+43.6
Cornea	Tears-anterior cornea	+5.2
Aqueous	Posterior cornea-aqueous	−5.8
Lens	Aqueous-anterior lens; lens core; posterior lens-vitreous	+19
	Total for Eye	**+62**

Important points obtained from Table 22-2 include:

o   The air-tear surface provides the greatest plus power to incident light rays (+43.6 D).

o   A dry cornea will produce blurry images.

o   The posterior cornea-aqueous surface provides minus power (−5.8 D).

o   The air, tears, and cornea together provide approximately 69.25% (+43 D) of the total refraction by the eye (+62 D).

o   Both surfaces of the crystalline lens provide plus power.

CLINICAL APPLICATIONS

BLURRING DUE TO DRY EYES

Experienced OMP know that patients with dry eyes complain of blurry vision. How is that explained?

As seen from information presented in Table 22-2, the greatest plus power in the eye is provided by the air-tear curved surface. When that surface is disrupted, a substantial amount of plus power (+43 D) is lost, resulting in blurring due to induced hyperopia. Blinking or instilling nonprescription artificial tears restores the curved surface and its powerful refraction. This may be a good remedy to follow when measuring refractive errors in older patients who frequently do not blink during refractometry.

Base Curve of Spectacle Lenses

Patients frequently complain of discomfort with a new pair of spectacles, even though lensometry, refractometry, and *pupillary distance* re-measurements indicate that every parameter is appropriate.[4]

In these cases, the base curve of the new spectacle lenses must be checked, and, if different from the current spectacle lenses, must be reordered with the base curve the patient used previously.

Refractive Power Changes During Diabetes Mellitus

Diabetes mellitus frequently results in 3 to 4 D of hyperopic and myopic shifts in refractive errors due to variations in *blood glucose*, which induce variations in the RI of the crystalline lens.[5]

Since the r of the anterior surface of the crystalline lens remains unchanged, the power changes result from changes in the value of n_2 when considering the aqueous-anterior lens curved surface:

$$P_{(D)} = \frac{(n_2 - n_1)}{r_{(m)}}$$

Higher blood glucose (mg/dL) = increase in n_2 = increase in $P_{(D)}$ = myopic shift
Lower blood glucose (mg/dL) = decrease in n_2 = decrease in $P_{(D)}$ = hyperopic shift

Refractive Surgery

Refractive surgery for eliminating, or at least reducing, myopia has been well established since radial keratotomy in the mid-20th century. Later advances led to many new procedures, and today, the worldwide population is familiar with the more common surgical procedures.[6]

The goal of refractive surgery for eliminating, or at least reducing, myopia is to increase the radius of curvature of the anterior cornea, thus reducing the positive vergence (plus power) of the air-tear-anterior cornea complex.

$$P_{(D)} = \frac{(n_2 - n_1)}{r_{(m)}}$$

Increase the $r_{(m)}$ = decrease the positive vergence = decrease the $P_{(D)}$

Methods for increasing the r include surgical procedures such as PRK, LASIK, LASEK, and INTACS.

Refractive surgery for eliminating, or at least reducing, hyperopia was established after successes in surgically treating myopia.

The goal of refractive surgery for eliminating, or at least reducing, hyperopia is to reduce the radius of curvature of the anterior cornea, thus increasing the positive vergence (plus power) of the air-tear-anterior cornea complex.

$$P_{(D)} = \frac{(n_2 - n_1)}{r_{(m)}}$$

Reduce the $r_{(m)}$ =   increase the positive vergence   =   increase the $P_{(D)}$

Methods for reducing the r include procedures such as LASIK, CK, and TK.

KERATOMETRY

Keratometry is the measurement of corneal curvatures, a procedure routinely performed by OMP. Although the keratometry readings are notated in power (D) in the patient chart, the power drum of an ophthalmometer (Keratometer) is also notated in radius of curvature (in mm). This is very useful because the base curve of a contact lens (see below) is typically notated in mm of r.

Power of the cornea (D) and its r (mm) are inversely related—when one increases, the other decreases. This relationship may be viewed on the power drum of an ophthalmometer that has notations in D and mm, both increasing in opposite directions.

CONTACT LENS BASE CURVE

Note: Standard textbooks should be consulted for reviewing the basics of contact lenses and their base curves.

The *base curve of contact lenses* is the *central posterior curve* of the contact lens, and this curve contacts the cornea. The base curve has a specific radius of curvature, which is based on the r of the cornea obtained by keratometry (see above).

Excessively flat-fitting (ie, loose) contact lenses move around too much on the cornea, producing a foreign body sensation and discomfort. These must be steepened (ie, tightened) by decreasing the base curve of the contact lenses.

As described above, the base curve is actually the r of the central posterior curve of the contact lens and may be mathematically expressed as:

$$P_{(D)} = \frac{(n_2 - n_1)}{r_{(m)}}$$

Where:

P = refractive power in D
n_1 = RI of the medium from which light is coming (first medium)
n_2 = RI of the medium into which light is going (second medium)
r = radius of curvature (in m) of refractive surface (base curve)

Thus, $r_{(m)}$, the base curve of the contact lens, may be changed to achieve an optical fit:

Decreasing $r_{(m)}$ of the base curve   =   steepens (ie, tightens) the contact lens

Excessively steep-fitting (ie, tight) contact lenses rest on the cornea too tightly, producing a burning sensation, a "hot-feeling" eye, redness, and discomfort. These must be flattened (ie, loosened) by increasing the base curve of the contact lenses.

As described above, the base curve is actually the r of the central posterior curve of the contact lens and may be mathematically expressed as:

$$P_{(D)} = \frac{(n_2 - n_1)}{r_{(m)}}$$

Where:

P = refractive power in D
n_1 = RI of the medium from which light is coming (first medium)

n_2 =   RI of the medium into which light is going (second medium)
r =   radius of curvature (in m) of refractive surface (base curve)

Thus, $r_{(m)}$, the base curve of the contact lens, may be changed to achieve an optical fit:

Increasing $r_{(m)}$ of the base curve   =   flattens (ie, loosens) the contact lens

Altering the base curves of SCL does not affect the prescription for correcting the refractive error. However, that is not the case when base curves of rigid gas-permeable (RGP) contact lenses are altered. When the RGP base curve is steepened, the refractive error correction must be changed in the minus direction (less plus or more minus). When the RGP base curve is flattened, the refractive error correction must be changed in the plus direction (more plus or less minus).

References

1. *Basic and Clinical Science Course, Section 3: Optics, Refraction, and Contact Lenses*. San Francisco, CA: American Academy of Ophthalmology; 1988.
2. Thall EH, Miller KM, Rosenthal P, Schechter RJ, Steinert RF, Beardsley TL. *Basic and Clinical Science Course, Section 3: Optics, Refraction, and Contact Lenses*. San Francisco, CA: American Academy of Ophthalmology; 2000.
3. Stein HA, Slatt BJ, Stein RM. *The Ophthalmic Assistant: A Guide for Ophthalmic Medical Personnel*. New York, NY: Mosby; 2000.
4. Shukla AV. Critical thinking protocols for ophthalmic medical personnel: refractometry. *J Ophthalmic Nursing & Technology*. 1999;18(1):24-28.
5. Thomas D, Graham EM. Ocular disorders associated with systemic diseases. In: Riordan-Eva P, Whitcher JP, eds. *Vaughan & Asbury's General Ophthalmology*. 17th ed. New York, NY: Lange/McGraw-Hill; 2008:305-339.
6. Weiss JS, Azar DT, Belin MW, et al. *Basic and Clinical Science Course, Section 14: Refractive Surgery*. San Francisco, CA: American Academy of Ophthalmology; 2004.

Review Questions

1.   The final variable described in considering refraction of light is:
     a.   refractive index
     b.   angle of incidence
     c.   radius of curvature
     d.   angle of refraction

2.   The formula for calculating the power of a curved surface may be rewritten as:
     a. $n_2 = [P_{(D)}]\,[r_{(m)}] + n_1$
     b. $r_{(m)} = \dfrac{(P_{(D)} - n_1)}{n_2}$
     c. $n_2 = [P_{(D)}]\,[r_{(m)}] - n_1$
     d. $r_{(m)} = \dfrac{(P_{(D)} - n_2)}{n_1}$

3. How will the power of a curved surface change if the diameter is changed from 1 m to 2 m, while all other factors remain unchanged?
    a. the power will decrease by half
    b. the power will stay unchanged
    c. the power will be zero
    d. the power will be doubled

4. How does the refractive power of the cornea change when it is applanated for intraocular pressure measurement?
    a. it will increase
    b. it will stay unchanged
    c. it will change unpredictably
    d. it will decrease

5. What is the power of a curved surface (RI = 1.200) of 20 cm diameter if light enters it after traveling through air?
    a. 5 D
    b. 2 D
    c. 10 D
    d. 20 D

6. How is the radius of curvature (r) of a curved surface affected if its power is reduced and the RI are unchanged?
    a. the r will increase
    b. the r will decrease
    c. the r will be unaffected
    d. the r should not be considered

7. A 54-year-old patient had cataract surgery, and a +20 D IOL was implanted. If this IOL (RI = 1.89) was held up in the air, its refractive power will most likely:
    a. remain unchanged
    b. decrease
    c. fluctuate
    d. increase

23

ACCOMMODATION

LEARNING Objectives

Upon completion of this chapter, the reader should be able to:

o describe changes in power of the crystalline lens.
o calculate the power of the distance correction for hyperopic children.
o calculate the power of the reading add for presbyopes.

Key Points

o Accommodation is the change in the focusing power of the crystalline lens.
o In children with high levels of hyperopia, accommodation may result in accommodative esotropia.
o The accommodative effort and response occur when an object is moved closer to the eye (ie, reading).
o With age, the accommodative response decreases, resulting in presbyopia and requiring bifocals for reading.
o Maximum focusing power of a normal crystalline lens focused at a distance is +19 D.
o Up to age 8, the maximum focusing power of a normal crystalline lens during accommodation is +33 D.
o Amplitude of accommodation is useful for determining the bifocal reading add power.
o Accommodation may be relaxed by using plus lenses.

ACCOMMODATION EFFORT AND RESPONSE

Accommodation is the change in the focusing power of the crystalline lens, and may be divided into two parts—*accommodative effort* and *accommodative response.*

Accommodative effort is the mechanism by which the *ciliary muscle* contracts and *zonules* relax in order to change the shape of the crystalline lens inside the eye. Accommodative response is the increase in focusing *power of the crystalline lens* due to an increase in convexity of the anterior surface of the crystalline lens to create sharp images.[1] During accommodation, the principle change in morphology occurs in the crystalline lens whose thickness (anterior-posterior distance) increases primarily by the anterior curved surface bowing forward. Accommodative response may be relaxed by using plus lenses.

In children who are high hyperopes, the accommodation effort and response may occur for distance visual acuity and will be enhanced when reading. Since accommodation is used for focusing a distant object on the fovea, additional accommodation will be required for reading. Because of the *synkinetic response* (reflex) (ie, accommodation, convergence, and *miosis* occurring together), the eyes may converge, resulting in *accommodative esotropia.* Such patients require a full hyperopic correction for distance and a bifocal for reading. Adding plus lenses for distance relaxes accommodation and eliminates accommodative esotropia.

In adults, the accommodative effort and response occurs when an object is moved closer to the eye (eg, reading). With age, the accommodative response decreases, resulting in presbyopia, and requires bifocals for reading. Pseudophakes retain the accommodative effort but no longer have the accommodative response.

When viewing at a distance, the following conditions apply to the lens and associated ocular structures:

o   ciliary muscle is relaxed

o   zonules are stretched

o   lens is thinnest

During accommodation, the following changes occur in the anatomy of the lens and associated ocular structures:

o   ciliary muscle contracts

o   zonules relax

o   lens thickens

Maximum power of a normal crystalline lens focused at a distance (ie, unaccommodating) is approximately +19 D. Of this, +9 D is provided by the curved anterior lens surface, and +10 D is provided by the curved posterior lens surface. Up to age 8, the maximum focusing power of a normal crystalline lens during accommodation is approximately +33 D. Thus, the lens can increase the focusing power by a maximum of +14 D (33 D – 19 D = 14 D).

CALCULATING THE AMPLITUDE OF ACCOMMODATION

Amplitude of accommodation (also termed *accommodative amplitude*) is the maximum change that can occur in the focusing power of the lens, and it decreases with increasing age. When bifocal add power is required for reading, the condition is termed *presbyopia* (typically starting at age 42), although the actual need for bifocal add power varies widely due to different reading distances and lighting conditions.[2]

As stated above, the maximum accommodative amplitude of a normal eye is +14 D when the lens changes its power from +19 D to +33 D. Maximum accommodative amplitude of a normal eye is present up to age 8, and it decreases after that according to the following generalized scheme[1]:

o Between ages 8 and 40, the accommodative amplitude decreases by +1 D every 4 years.

o At age 40, the remaining accommodative amplitude is +6 D.

o Between ages 40 and 48, the accommodative amplitude decreases by +1.5 D every 4 years.

o At age 48, the remaining accommodative amplitude is +3 D.

o Above age 48, accommodative amplitude decreases by +0.5 D every 4 years.

o Accommodative amplitude is 0 at age 72.

The amplitude of accommodation may be determined using the scheme above or calculated using the following formulae:

Age 8 to 39:   amplitude $= 14 - \frac{(age - 8)}{4}$

Age 40 to 48:   amplitude $= 6 - \{1.5\,[\frac{(age - 40)}{4}]\}$

Age >48:   amplitude $= 3 - \{0.5\,[\frac{(age - 48)}{4}]\}$

OPTICAL RELATIONSHIPS AND DEFINITIONS

The amplitude of accommodation can be optically defined as the difference between the *far point* and *near point* of the eye:

The far point (f) is the farthest point (in m) at which an object is in focus. The far point is also the refractive error (F), and may be converted to diopters (D):

$$F_{(D)} = \frac{1}{f_{(m)}}$$

For convenience, cm or mm may also be used:

$$F_{(D)} = \frac{100}{f_{(cm)}} = \frac{1000}{f_{(mm)}}$$

F will be minus if the far point is in minus space, or in front of the eye (eg, myopes), and positive if it is in plus space, or behind the eye (eg, hyperopes).

The near point (n) is the closest point (in m) at which an object is in focus, and occurs when the lens is maximally accommodating (N). It may be converted to D:

$$N_{(D)} = \frac{1}{n_{(m)}}$$

For convenience, cm or mm may also be used:

$$N_{(D)} = \frac{100}{n_{(cm)}} = \frac{1000}{n_{(mm)}}$$

In corrected or uncorrected emmetropes, N depends on the available accommodative amplitude.

Example 1

What is the near point of a 20-year-old emmetrope or corrected emmetrope?

The amplitude of accommodation may be determined using age and the scheme described above:

Age 8 to 39:

$$\text{amplitude} = 14 - \frac{(\text{age} - 8)}{4}$$

$$\text{amplitude} = 14 - \frac{(20 - 8)}{4}$$

$$\text{amplitude} = 14 - \frac{12}{4}$$

$$\text{amplitude} = 14 - 3$$

$$\text{amplitude} = 11 \text{ D}$$

Converting to distance:

$$N_{(D)} = \frac{1}{n_{(m)}}$$

$$n_{(m)} = \frac{1}{N_{(D)}}$$

$$n_{(m)} = \frac{1}{11}$$

$$n_{(m)} = 0.09 \text{ m}$$

$$n_{(m)} = 9 \text{ cm}$$

The near point will be at 9 cm, and objects closer than that will appear blurry.

In uncorrected myopes, the far point (F) will be in minus space in front of the eye (eg, at 25 cm for a −4 D myope) and the near point (N) will be correspondingly closer, depending on the available accommodative amplitude (A).

$$N = A + F$$

Example 2

What is the near point of a 28-year-old who has 4 D of uncorrected myopia?

The amplitude of accommodation may be determined using age and the scheme described above:

Age 8 to 39:

$$\text{amplitude} = 14 - \frac{(\text{age} - 8)}{4}$$

$$\text{amplitude} = 14 - \frac{(28 - 8)}{4}$$

$$\text{amplitude} = 14 - \frac{20}{4}$$

$$\text{amplitude} = 14 - 5$$

$$\text{amplitude} = 9 \text{ D}$$

Since:

$$N = A + F$$
$$N = 9 + 4$$
$$N = 13\ D$$

Converting to distance:

$$N_{(D)} = \frac{1}{n_{(m)}}$$

$$n_{(m)} = \frac{1}{N_{(D)}}$$

$$n_{(m)} = \frac{1}{13}$$

$$n_{(m)} = 0.07\ m$$
$$n_{(m)} = 7\ cm$$

The near point will be at 7 cm, and objects closer than that will appear blurry.

In uncorrected hyperopes the near point (N) will recede farther in front of the eye because part of the available accommodative amplitude (A) will be used to correct the hyperopia. Thus, in hyperopes, the near point will be the difference between A and the far point (uncorrected refractive error; F):

$$N = A - F$$

Example 3

What is the near point of a 32-year-old who has 5 D of uncorrected hyperopia?
The amplitude of accommodation may be determined using age and the scheme described above:

Age 8 to 39:

$$\text{amplitude} = 14 - \frac{(age - 8)}{4}$$

$$\text{amplitude} = 14 - \frac{(32 - 8)}{4}$$

$$\text{amplitude} = 14 - \frac{24}{4}$$

$$\text{amplitude} = 14 - 6$$
$$\text{amplitude} = 8\ D$$

Since:

$$N = A - F$$
$$N = 8 - (+5)$$
$$N = 8 - 5$$
$$N = 3\ D$$

Converting to distance:

$$N_{(D)} = \frac{1}{n_{(m)}}$$

$$n_{(m)} = \frac{1}{N_{(D)}}$$

$$n_{(m)} = \frac{1}{3}$$

$$n_{(m)} = 0.33 \text{ m}$$
$$n_{(m)} = 33 \text{ cm}$$

The near point will be at 33 cm, and objects closer than that will appear blurry.

MEASURING THE AMPLITUDE OF ACCOMMODATION

During accommodation, the far point moves closer to the eye, and the near point also moves correspondingly closer. As described above, accommodative effort is the contraction of the ciliary muscle, while accommodative response is the increase in power of the crystalline lens.[1] During presbyopia, the accommodative effort remains intact, but the response progressively diminishes.

Accommodative response of the eye is expressed in two ways:

1. Amplitude of accommodation (change of power in D), which is useful for determining the reading add power.

2. Range of accommodation (distance between far and near points of the eye), which is useful for assessing the ability to perform a task at near.

Amplitude of accommodation is a monocular function. Binocular amplitudes will be greater than monocular amplitudes. Thus, patients can read finer print with both eyes than with each eye individually.[1]

It is frequently necessary to make two measurements: 1) the accommodative need, in which the distance that a near task is performed is converted to D; and 2) the average of monocular amplitudes of accommodation.

Table 23-1			
Task	Accommodative Need*	Average Monocular Amplitude	Bifocal Add Power (amplitude minus diopters required)
Reading at 33 cm	+3 D	+4 D	+1 D
Needlework at 20 cm	+5 D		+3 D

*Distance at which a near task is performed, converted to D.

An example is a 44-year-old corrected emmetrope who likes to do needlework at 20 cm compared to reading at 33 cm (Table 23-1).

Monocular amplitude of accommodation may be measured two ways[1]:

1. the Prince Rule (metal rod with inches, cm, m, D, and a *Reichert Nearpoint Rotochart*)

2. spherical lenses

PRINCE RULE

o   The Prince Rule is properly positioned on the refractor (Phoroptor).

o   The OS is occluded, and a +3 D spherical lens is inserted before the OD.

o   This brings the far point to 33 cm and the near point correspondingly closer.

o   Patient views J2 or J3 print on a Reichert Nearpoint Rotochart.

o   The Reichert Nearpoint Rotochart is first moved farther away, and the D are noted for the position where the print first appears blurry. This is the far point.

o   Then, the Reichert Nearpoint Rotochart is moved closer, and the D are noted for the position where the print first appears blurry. This is the near point.

o   The difference in D between the far and near points is the monocular amplitude of accommodation for the OD.

o   Repeat process with the OS.

Spherical Lenses

o   The Prince Rule is properly positioned on the refractor (Phoroptor).

o   The OS is occluded, and the patient uses OD to view J2 or J3 on a Reichert Nearpoint Rotochart, positioned at 40 cm.

o   Accommodation is stimulated by adding minus spherical lenses, and the D are noted when the print first appears blurry. This is the far point.

o   Then, accommodation is relaxed by adding plus spherical lenses, and the D are noted when the print first appears blurry. This is the near point.

o   The difference in D between the far and near points is the monocular amplitude of accommodation for the OD.

o   Repeat process with the OS.

Accommodation and the Synkinetic Response

When the eyes, initially focused at a distance, attempt to focus at a near task such as reading, the following physiologic changes take place and are together termed the *synkinetic response (reflex):*

o   eyes accommodate

o   eyes converge

o   pupils constrict (miosis)

Frequently, the distance refractive error is so hyperopic that accommodation is used to provide the needed plus power for distance. The greater the hyperopia, the greater the accommodative effort for distance. In this condition, the eyes may also converge due to the synkinetic response, thus producing esotropia, which will be enhanced when the patient focuses at near. Since accommodation is used to produce the esotropia, such deviations are termed *accommodative esotropia.* Since refractive errors in children are typically hyperopic, accommodative esotropia is frequently seen in children, but may also occur in adults.

Hyperopic children with accommodative esotropia wear spectacle lenses with the distance correction, as well as a bifocal reading add whose goal is to relax accommodation when performing near tasks such as reading. Since plus power is provided by spectacle lenses for distance and near, accommodation is relaxed and the esotropia is eliminated.

The protocol for determining the distance correction in children with isometropic hyperopia is:

o   Determine the true hyperopia by cycloplegic refractometry.

o   Determine the available amplitude of accommodation.

o   Divide the accommodative amplitude by 2.

o   Keep one-half in reserve.

o   The other half may be used for accommodating for distance viewing.

o   Distance correction becomes:

$$(\text{Refractive error}) - \frac{(\text{Accommodative amplitude})}{2}$$

o   If the result is in minus, no correction is required.

Example 4

A 12-year-old patient whose cycloplegic refractometry result is +5 SPH OU:

$$
\begin{aligned}
\text{Cycloplegic refractometry} \ &= \ \text{+5 SPH} \\
\text{Amplitude of accommodation} \ &= \ (+14) - (+1) \\
&= \ +14 - 1 \\
&= \ +13
\end{aligned}
$$

$$
\text{Divide the accommodative amplitude by 2} \ = \ \frac{+13}{2}
$$

$$
\begin{aligned}
&= \ +6.5 \\
\text{Keep one-half in reserve} \ &= \ +6.5 \\
\text{Use other half:} \ &= \ +6.5
\end{aligned}
$$

$$
\begin{aligned}
\text{Distance correction is} \ &= \ (\text{Refractive error}) - \frac{(\text{Accommodative amplitude})}{2} \\
&= \ (+5) - (+6.5) \\
&= \ +5 - 6.5 \\
&= \ -1.5
\end{aligned}
$$

Since the result is in minus, no correction is required, although licensed practitioners may choose to give some plus power to prevent accommodative esotropia.

Example 5

A 12-year-old patient whose cycloplegic refractometry result is +7.5 SPH OU:

$$
\begin{aligned}
\text{Cycloplegic refractometry} \ &= \ \text{+7.5 SPH} \\
\text{Amplitude of accommodation} \ &= \ (+14) - (+1) \\
&= \ +14 - 1 \\
&= \ +13
\end{aligned}
$$

$$
\text{Divide the accommodative amplitude by 2} \ = \ \frac{+13}{2}
$$

$$
\begin{aligned}
&= \ +6.5 \\
\text{Keep one-half in reserve} \ &= \ +6.5 \\
\text{Use other half:} \ &= \ +6.5
\end{aligned}
$$

$$
\begin{aligned}
\text{Distance correction is} \ &= \ (\text{Refractive error}) - \frac{(\text{Accommodative amplitude})}{2} \\
&= \ (+7.5) - (+6.5) \\
&= \ +7.5 - 6.5 \\
&= \ +1
\end{aligned}
$$

Distance correction is +1 SPH OU. The patient requires +7.5 D, of which +1 D is provided by spectacle lenses, and +6.5 D by accommodation. Licensed practitioners may choose to give additional plus power to decrease the +6.5 D provided by accommodation and prevent accommodative esotropia.

Spectacle lenses for correcting anisometropia in hyperopic children are balanced by applying accommodative amplitude to the amount of hyperopia in each eye. In this scheme, both eyes are allowed to accommodate using half of the available accommodative amplitude. This provides some of the needed plus power OU. Spectacle lenses are then recommended for the remaining amount of uncorrected hyperopia in each hyperopic eye.

Protocol for determining the distance correction in children with anisometropic hyperopia is:

o   Determine the true hyperopia by cycloplegic refractometry.

o   Determine the available monocular amplitude of accommodation.

o   Divide accommodative amplitude by 2.

o   Keep one-half in reserve.

o   The other half may be used for accommodating at distance.

o   Distance correction for each eye is:

$$\text{(Refractive error of hyperopic eye)} - \frac{\text{(Accommodative amplitude)}}{2}$$

Example 6

A 6-year-old patient whose cycloplegic refractometry is OD +8.00 SPH and OS +10.00 SPH:

$$
\begin{aligned}
\text{Amplitude of accommodation} \ &= \ (+14) - (0) \\
&= \ +14 \\
\text{Divide the accommodative amplitude by 2} \ &= \ \frac{+14}{2} \\
&= \ +7 \\
\text{Keep one-half in reserve} \ &= \ +7 \\
\text{Use other half:} \ &= \ +7
\end{aligned}
$$

$$
\begin{aligned}
\text{Distance correction for OD is} \ &= \ \text{(Refractive error)} - \frac{\text{(Accommodative amplitude)}}{2} \\
&= \ (+8) - (+7) \\
&= \ +8 - 7 \\
&= \ +1 \text{ D}
\end{aligned}
$$

$$
\begin{aligned}
\text{Distance correction for OS is} \ &= \ \text{(Refractive error)} - \frac{\text{(Accommodative amplitude)}}{2} \\
&= \ (+10) - (+7) \\
&= \ +10 - 7 \\
&= \ +3 \text{ D}
\end{aligned}
$$

Spectacle lens correction is:

OD: +1.00 SPH

OS: +3.00 SPH

The patient needs +8.00 SPH for the OD. Of that, +1 D is provided by a spectacle lens, and +7 D by accommodation. The patient needs +10.00 SPH for the OS. Of that, +3 D is provided by a spectacle lens, and +7 D by accommodation. Licensed practitioners may give additional plus power OU.

ACCOMMODATION AND READING ADD POWER

Having set the stage, we can now investigate how lens corrections are considered for presbyopia. The concepts are very similar to those described above. The only additional parameter needed is accommodative need, which is the dioptric value of the distance at which the near task is performed:

$$\text{Accommodative need}_{(D)} = \frac{1}{\text{Distance}_{(m)}}$$

For the sake of convenience, cm or mm may also be used:

$$\text{Accommodative need}_{(D)} = \frac{100}{\text{Distance}_{(cm)}} = \frac{1000}{\text{Distance}_{(mm)}}$$

If a patient reads at 33 cm, then the accommodative need is +3 D:

$$\text{Accommodative need}_{(D)} = \frac{100}{\text{Distance}_{(cm)}} = \frac{100}{33} = 3$$

Or, if a patient does needlework at 20 cm, then the accommodative need is +5 D:

$$\text{Accommodative need}_{(D)} = \frac{100}{\text{Distance}_{(cm)}} = \frac{100}{20} = 5$$

The general protocol is[1]:
o   Determine accommodative need (D).
o   Determine the available amplitude of accommodation (D).
o   Divide amplitude of accommodation by 2.
o   Keep one-half in reserve.
o   The other half may be used for accommodation at near.
o   Reading add is:

$$(\text{Accommodative need}) - \frac{(\text{Accommodative amplitude})}{2}$$

Example 7

Determine the reading add power for a 44-year-old first-time presbyope who reads at 25 cm.

$$
\begin{aligned}
\text{Accommodative need} \ &= \ 25 \text{ cm} \\
&= \ \frac{100}{25} \\
&= \ +4 \text{ D} \\
\text{Amplitude of accommodation} \ &= \ 6 - \{1.5 \,[\tfrac{(age - 40)}{4}]\} \\
&= \ 6 - \{1.5 \,[\tfrac{(44 - 40)}{4}]\} \\
&= \ 6 - \{1.5 \,[\tfrac{(4)}{4}]\} \\
&= \ 6 - 1.5 \\
&= \ +4.5 \\
\text{Divide amplitude of accommodation by 2} \ &= \ \frac{4.5}{2} \\
&= \ +2.25 \text{ D} \\
\text{Keep one-half in reserve} \ &= \ +2.25 \text{ D} \\
\text{The other half may be used for} \\
\text{accommodation at near} \ &= \ +2.25 \text{ D}
\end{aligned}
$$

$$
\begin{aligned}
\text{Reading add is} \ &= \ (\text{Accommodative need}) - \frac{(\text{Accommodative amplitude})}{2} \\
&= \ (4) - \frac{(4.5)}{2} \\
&= \ 4 - 2.25 \\
&= \ +1.75 \text{ D}
\end{aligned}
$$

A +1.75 D reading add will be required.

References

1. Thall EH, Miller KM, Rosenthal P, Schechter RJ, Steinert RF, Beardsley TL. *Basic and Clinical Science Course, Section 3: Optics, Refraction, and Contact Lenses.* San Francisco, CA: American Academy of Ophthalmology; 2000.
2. Stein HA, Stein RM, Freeman MI. *The Ophthalmic Assistant: A Text for Allied and Associated Ophthalmic Personnel.* 8th ed. Chicago, IL: Mosby; 2006.

Review Questions

1. Accommodative effort refers to the:
    a. contraction of zonules
    b. contraction of the anterior capsule
    c. relaxation of the ciliary muscle
    d. contraction of the ciliary muscle

2. Accommodative response refers to the:
    a. increase in zonule length
    b. increase in anterior lens capsule convexity
    c. relaxation of the ciliary muscle
    d. increase in lens density

3. In maximum accommodation, the power of the lens changes from:
    a. +62 D to +76 D
    b. +19 D to +33 D
    c. +19 D to +50 D
    d. +12 D to +62 D

4. Accommodation can be relaxed by providing a patient with a:
    a. PL lens
    b. minus lens
    c. prism
    d. plus lens

5. During maximum accommodation by a 7-year-old, the total power of the eye is (assume that the total power of a normal eye is +62 D when no accommodation is used):
    a. +76 D
    b. +62 D
    c. +33 D
    d. +19 D

24

REFRACTIVE ERRORS

LEARNING Objectives

Upon completion of this chapter, the reader should be able to:

o   describe hyperopia, myopia, and types of astigmatism.
o   calculate powers for latent, manifest, and absolute hyperopia.
o   describe lens corrections for astigmatism.

KEY POINTS

o   Emmetropic eyes have the appropriate amount of plus power and do not require any refractive correction.
o   Ametropic eyes do not have the appropriate amount of plus power and require refractive correction.
o   Ametropia includes myopia, hyperopia, and astigmatism.
o   Refractometry is the process of measuring a refractive error using optical principles.
o   Refraction is the process of making a clinical decision for prescribing corrective lenses.
o   Myopia, or nearsightedness, occurs in eyes that have excessive plus power.
o   Hyperopia, or farsightedness, occurs in eyes that have inadequate plus power.
o   Children with moderate hyperopia can correct most hyperopic errors.
o   Hyperopia is classified as latent, manifest, and absolute.
o   The general rule is: absolute hyperopic correction (required); manifest hyperopic correction (may be given); and latent hyperopic correction (must not be given).

KEY POINTS (CONTINUED)

o   Regular astigmatism may be of five types: simple myopic, simple hyperopic, compound myopic, compound hyperopic, and mixed astigmatism.

o   If the vertical axis is steeper, the astigmatism is termed *with-the-rule* (or W/R).

o   If the horizontal axis is steeper, the astigmatism is termed *against-the-rule* (or A/R).

o   Irregular astigmatism results when the corneal topography is altered in such a way that it cannot be corrected by spectacle lenses.

REFRACTIVE ERRORS—INTRODUCTION AND DEFINITIONS

Determining the refractive error can distinguish between visual loss due to an organic disease versus *uncorrected refractive error*. All patients whose best corrected visual acuity is worse than 20/20 should be measured for refractive errors.[1,2]

Many terms are used to describe various conditions related to refraction in the eye.

In emmetropia, light rays from infinity are focused on the fovea and produce a sharp image. Emmetropic eyes have the appropriate amount of plus power and do not require any refractive correction. Patients who are fully corrected with lenses are commonly termed *corrected emmetropes*.

In ametropia, light rays from infinity do not focus on the fovea and produce a blurry image. Ametropic eyes do not have the appropriate amount of plus power and require refractive correction. Ametropia includes:

o   myopia

o   hyperopia

o   astigmatism

Refractometry is the process of measuring a refractive error using optical principles. This is commonly termed *manifest refraction* (MR), although the correct term should be *manifest refractometry*. An MR may be performed by trained ophthalmic medical personnel (OMP) using a refractor (Phoroptor), retinoscope, trial lenses, or automated instruments.

Refraction is the process of making a clinical decision for prescribing corrective lenses using information from refractometry, visual acuity, accommodative ability, muscle balance, and lens clarity. Refraction requires medical decision making and clinical judgment, and may only be performed by licensed ophthalmologists (MDs and DOs) and optometrists (ODs).

MYOPIA

Myopia, or *nearsightedness*, occurs in eyes that have excessive plus power. Therefore, the sharpest image forms anterior to the fovea. The far point of myopic eyes is in plus space and corresponds to the un-accommodative spectacle lens correction:

For example,

- o A –1.00 SPH myope will have the far point located at 100 cm.
- o A –3.00 SPH myope will have the far point located at 33.3 cm.

Squinting is a typical response by myopes because it improves uncorrected visual acuity by creating a pinhole effect, in which the central rays are incident at 90 degrees and do not require refraction. However, constant squinting may lead to headaches and asthenopia. In addition, squinting has the potential of decreasing the extent of a normal visual field.

Myopia may be due to various causes[3]:

- o Axial myopia: The axial length of the myopic eye is greater than normal, causing parallel light rays to focus anterior to the retina. Axial myopia is the most common type of myopia.
- o Curvature myopia: The eye has normal axial length, but the cornea is steeper than normal with a radius of curvature less than normal, causing parallel light rays to focus anterior to the retina.
- o Index myopia: The refractive index (RI) of the lens increases, thus causing parallel light rays to focus anterior to the retina. Index myopia may be caused by diabetes mellitus and cataracts.

Symptoms of myopia are classic and include:

- o Uncorrected distance vision is blurry.
- o Uncorrected near vision is clear.

Myopia should be fully corrected to permit clear distance vision. Since minus lenses reduce image size, corrections greater than –4 D produce smaller-sized images on the retina, and this effect increases with greater powers. Therefore, depth perception may also be affected since smaller retinal images are perceived by the brain to be at greater distances.

Retinal image size decreases (therefore, difficulties in depth perception) and may be minimized by using contact lenses, which do not affect image sizes to the same extent as spectacle lenses. Contact lenses also do not have aberrations produced by peripheries of thick spectacle lenses, thus providing better peripheral vision.

HYPEROPIA

Hyperopia, or *farsightedness*, occurs in eyes that have inadequate plus power. The sharpest image will form posterior to the fovea. The far point of hyperopic eyes is in minus space and beyond infinity. The sharpest image must be moved anteriorly on to the fovea. This may be accomplished in two ways:

1. Using accommodation to provide plus power.
2. Using plus lenses to provide additional plus power.

Hyperopia may be due to various causes[3]:

- o Axial hyperopia: The axial length of the hyperopic eye is shorter than normal, causing parallel light rays to focus posterior to the fovea.
- o Curvature hyperopia: The eye has normal axial length, but the cornea is flatter than normal with a radius of curvature greater than normal, causing parallel light rays to focus posterior to the retina.

Children with moderate hyperopia do not have any symptoms since their ample accommodative amplitude can correct most hyperopic errors.[4] However, children with great amounts of hyperopia may converge and would then require special attention for their hyperopia. A general rule of thumb for children is:

$$\text{Hyperopic correction} = \text{CR spherical portion} - \frac{\text{(Accommodative amplitude)}}{2}$$

In adults, symptoms of hyperopia generally reveal themselves when performing close tasks (eg, reading), and may include:

o headaches

o burning sensation

o pulling sensation

o diplopia

All of these symptoms result from the constant need to accommodate. In a patient of presbyopic age (phakic patients, 42 years old and older), symptoms manifest themselves when the near point recedes beyond the length of the patient's arm.

Hyperopia is classified as latent, manifest, and absolute (Table 24-1).[3]

Table 24-1			
Type of Hyperopia	**Definition**	**Uncorrected Visual Acuity**	**Spectacle Lens Correction**
Latent	Corrected by accommodation	Normal	No plus lens needed (they will cause blurring)
Manifest (facultative)	Corrected by accommodation or by plus lenses	Normal	Plus lenses may be used but are not necessary
Absolute	Corrected by plus lenses only	Blurry	Plus lenses necessary

The best way to think about correcting the various types of hyperopia is to investigate how the sharpest images may be moved on to the fovea. Recall that hyperopia occurs in eyes that have inadequate positive vergence (plus power). Thus, the sharpest image would form posterior to the fovea. To correct any type of hyperopia, the image simply needs to be moved anteriorly to the fovea by somehow providing plus power (Figure 24-1):

o In latent hyperopia, the crystalline lens provides plus power. Since this plus power is always present, no plus lenses are required to move the image anteriorly.

o In manifest (facultative) hyperopia, accommodation can provide plus power. Plus lenses or accommodation are required to move the image anteriorly.

o In absolute hyperopia, plus lenses are required to move the image anteriorly.

Absolute hyperopia may be measured, and it represents the plus power required to first achieve best corrected visual acuity (eg, +2 D required to first read, say, 20/25^{+2}). Manifest (facultative) hyperopia may be measured, and represents the additional plus power required to maintain best corrected visual acuity (eg, an additional +1 D required to continue reading 20/25^{+2}). Latent hyperopia must be calculated and requires cycloplegic refractometry (see Figure 24-1).

Latent hyperopia (L) = Cycloplegic refractometry (CR) – [Absolute (A) + Manifest hyperopia (M)]

$$L = CR - (A + M)$$

The general rule is[3]:

Absolute hyperopic correction:	Required
Manifest hyperopic correction:	May be corrected to relax accommodation
Latent hyperopic correction:	Not required

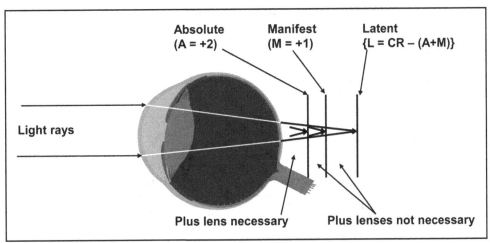

Figure 24-1. Types of hyperopia. The latent (L) and manifest (M) components of hyperopia do not require correction since accommodation moves the images anteriorly on the fovea. The absolute hyperopia (A) component does not use accommodation and requires a plus lens to move the image on the fovea. (CR is cycloplegic refractometry.)

Example 1

See Figure 24-1 for details.

$$
\begin{aligned}
\text{Absolute hyperopia (A)} &= +2 \quad \text{(patient first reads } 20/25^{+2}) \\
\text{Manifest hyperopia (M)} &= +1 \quad \text{(patient continues to read } 20/25^{+2}) \\
\text{Cycloplegic refractometry (CR)} &= +5 \\
\text{Latent hyperopia (L)} &= CR - (A + M) \\
L &= +5 - (+2 + 1) \\
L &= +5 - (+3) \\
L &= +5 - 3 \\
L &= +2
\end{aligned}
$$

This patient requires +2 D to read $20/25^{+2}$ and may be corrected with an additional +1 D to relax accommodation, but does not require the full cycloplegic correction (+5 D).

So, what will happen to the refraction in a patient's eye if the full cycloplegic hyperopia is corrected?

In Example 1, the patient requires +2 D, but may be corrected with an additional +1 D, making it +3 D total. If the patient is corrected with +5 D instead, then after the cycloplegic effects wear off, the patient's latent hyperopia of +2 D will be triggered, and the patient will have excess plus power, thus inducing myopia and blurring. Even if the patient relaxes the manifest (facultative) hyperopia equal to +1 D, there will still be an excess plus power, creating blurring due to induced myopia.

Example 2

Determine the various hyperopic components in the following patient and the power of the distance correction:

$$
\begin{aligned}
\text{Patient age} &= \text{7-year-old patient} \\
\text{Uncorrected visual acuity} &= 20/40 \\
\text{Visual acuity corrects to } 20/20+2 &= +3 \text{ D} \\
\text{Visual acuity still } 20+2 &= +4 \text{ D} \\
\text{Cycloplegic refractometry} &= +6 \text{ D} \\
\text{Amplitude of accommodation} & \\
\text{(see Chapter 23)} &= +14 \text{ D} \\
\text{Half of the accommodative} & \\
\text{amplitude can be used} &= +7
\end{aligned}
$$

Condition	Result
Absolute Hyperopia	+3 D
Manifest (Facultative) Hyperopia	$= (+4) - (+3)$ $= +4 - 3$ $= +1$ D
Latent Hyperopia	$= (+6) - (+3 + 1)$ $= (+6) - (+4)$ $= +6 - 4$ $= +2$ D
Power of the Distance Correction	None

Since the patient can use up to +7 D of accommodative amplitude, no correction is required.

Example 3

Determine the various hyperopic components in the following patient, and the power of the distance correction:

$$
\begin{aligned}
\text{Patient age} &= \text{36-year-old patient} \\
\text{Uncorrected visual acuity} &= 20/70 \\
\text{Visual acuity corrects to } 20/20+2 &= +5 \text{ D} \\
\text{Visual acuity still } 20+2 &= +6 \text{ D} \\
\text{Cycloplegic refractometry} &= +7 \text{ D} \\
\text{Amplitude of accommodation} & \\
\text{(see Chapter 23)} &= +14 - \frac{(36 - 8)}{4} \\
&= +14 - \frac{(+28)}{4} \\
&= +14 - (+7) \\
&= +14 - 7 \\
&= +7 \\
\text{Half of the accommodative} & \\
\text{amplitude can be used} &= +3.50
\end{aligned}
$$

Condition	Result
Absolute Hyperopia	+5 D
Manifest (Facultative) Hyperopia	= (+6) – (+5) = +6 – 5 = +1 D
Latent Hyperopia	= (+7) – (+5 + 1) = (+7) – (+6) = +7 – 6 = +1 D
Power of the Distance Correction	= (+5) – (+3.50) = +5 – 3.50 = +1.50 D Patient needs +5 D. Of this, +1.50 D is provided by spectacle lenses and +3.50 D by accommodation. Patient may be given an additional +1 D to relax accommodation. Distance correction then becomes +2.50 D.

This patient requires +1.5 D to read 20/20[+2] and may be corrected with an additional +1 D to relax accommodation, but must not be corrected with the full cycloplegic correction (+7 D).

REGULAR ASTIGMATISM

In astigmatism, light rays do not refract equally in all meridians and do not focus equally in all meridians. Due to unequal focusing, light comes to a focus along a line instead of a point (astigma = no point).

Astigmatism may be regular or irregular. Whereas regular astigmatism (caused by refraction, as described above) is correctable by spectacle and contact lenses, irregular astigmatism (caused by corneal irregularities) is not correctable by spectacle and soft contact lenses (SCL), and requires rigid gas-permeable (RGP) contact lenses or corneal surgery.

Since the most common type of astigmatism seen in clinical settings is regular astigmatism, this will be discussed ahead.

The concepts of Conoid of Sturm and the Circle of Least Confusion have direct applications in considering regular astigmatism, and readers are encouraged to see Chapter 20 for those details.

Regular astigmatism may be corrected using cylindrical and spherocylindrical lenses.[4] In regular astigmatism, the axes of maximum and minimum powers are at 90 degrees to each other, and are separated by the Conoid of Sturm. Regular astigmatism may be of five types (see Chapters 8, 17, and 18 for details):

1. simple myopic astigmatism
2. simple hyperopic astigmatism
3. compound myopic astigmatism
4. compound hyperopic astigmatism
5. mixed astigmatism

Regular astigmatism may be caused by the cornea and/or the crystalline lens because the radius of curvature (in mm), and, therefore, power (in D), is not equal in all directions. If the vertical axis is steeper, the astigmatism is termed *with-the-rule* (or W/R). If the horizontal axis is steeper, the astigmatism is termed *against-the-rule* (or A/R). W/R corneal astigmatism is more common, whereas the crystalline lens generally causes A/R astigmatism.

Regular astigmatism, as measured during refractometry, is the total astigmatism (AT), and is the sum of corneal astigmatism (AK) and lens (lenticular) astigmatism (AL):

$$(AT) = (AK) + (AL)$$

Patients with uncorrected astigmatism cannot see clearly at a distance or near, and will typically squint to eliminate one set of light rays. Reading material might be held very close to take advantage of magnification. The net result of all of these adaptations is that uncorrected astigmatism causes brow aches.[5]

Example 4

Identify the source(s) and type(s) of regular astigmatism with the following parameters:

Keratometry	=	42.50 @ 165 / 44.00 @ 75
AK	=	1.5 D W/R
Manifest refractometry	=	−3.25 +1.50 x 75
AT	=	1.5 D W/R
AT	=	(AK) + (AL)
AL	=	(AT) − (AK)
AL	=	(1.5) − (1.5)
AL	=	0

The 1.5 D of regular astigmatism is corneal, and the axis (75) indicates W/R.

Example 5

Identify the source(s) and type(s) of regular astigmatism with the following parameters:

Keratometry	=	44.50 / 44.50
AK	=	0
Manifest refractometry	=	+1.25 +1.00 x 165
AT	=	1 D A/R
AT	=	(AK) + (AL)
AL	=	(AT) − (AK)
AL	=	(1) − (0)
AL	=	1

The 1 D of regular astigmatism is lenticular, and the axis (165) indicates A/R.

Example 6

Identify the source(s) and type(s) of regular astigmatism with the following parameters:

Keratometry	=	42.50 @ 165 / 44.00 @ 75
AK	=	1.5 D W/R
Manifest refractometry	=	+1.25 SPH
AT	=	0

$$
\begin{aligned}
AT &= (AK) + (AL) \\
AL &= (AT) - (AK) \\
AL &= (0) - (1.5) \\
AL &= -1.5
\end{aligned}
$$

The 1.5 D of regular astigmatism is lenticular and A/R (ie, at 90 degrees to corneal astigmatism). The total astigmatism is 0 because the 1 D W/R corneal astigmatism is canceled by 1 D A/R lenticular astigmatism.

References

1. Shukla AV. Critical thinking protocols for ophthalmic medical personnel: importance of pinhole visual acuity and refractometry. *Viewpoints, Association of Technical Personnel in Ophthalmology.* 2006;September.
2. Shukla AV. Critical thinking protocols for ophthalmic medical personnel: testing for blurry vision. *Viewpoints, Association of Technical Personnel in Ophthalmology.* 2007;March.
3. Stein HA, Stein RM, Freeman MI. *The Ophthalmic Assistant: A Text for Allied and Associated Ophthalmic Personnel.* 8th ed. Chicago, IL: Mosby; 2006.
4. Thall EH, Miller KM, Rosenthal P, Schechter RJ, Steinert RF, Beardsley TL. *Basic and Clinical Science Course, Section 3: Optics, Refraction, and Contact Lenses.* San Francisco, CA: American Academy of Ophthalmology; 2000.
5. Shukla AV. Critical thinking protocols for ophthalmic medical personnel: refractometry. *J Ophthalmic Nursing & Technology.* 1999;18(1):24-28.

Review Questions

1. The condition in which the eye does not have the appropriate amount of plus power is:
   a. myopia
   b. ametropia
   c. hyperopia
   d. emmetropia

2. Changes in the plus power of the eye due to a decrease in the radius of curvature of the cornea are typically seen in:
   a. myopia
   b. ametropia
   c. hyperopia
   d. emmetropia

3. Accommodation is frequently used to produce a sharp image of a distant object in:
   a. myopia
   b. ametropia
   c. hyperopia
   d. emmetropia

4. A patient who first sees 20/20 with +2.00 D and continues to see 20/20 with an additional +0.75 D:
    a. must be given +2.75 D
    b. must be given +0.75 D
    c. may be given +2.75 D
    d. may be given +0.75 D

5. A patient who first sees 20/20 with +1.00 D, continues to see 20/20 with an additional +0.75 D, and whose cycloplegic refractometry is +3.50 D:
    a. must be given +3.50 D
    b. must be given +0.75 D
    c. may be given +1. 75 D
    d. may be given +3.50 D

6. A 65-year-old patient whose preoperative manifest refractometry was +2.00 SPH had unremarkable cataract surgery with a posterior chamber intraocular lens implant. Postoperative refractometry was −0.50 +1.50 x 87. These data indicate the presence of:
    a. 1.5 D of A/R postop corneal astigmatism
    b. 1.5 D of A/R preop lenticular astigmatism
    c. 0.5 D of W/R postop corneal astigmatism
    d. 1.5 D of W/R preop lenticular astigmatism

25

PRENTICE'S RULE, DECENTRATION, AND INDUCED PRISM

LEARNING OBJECTIVES

Upon completion of this chapter, the reader should be able to:

o   describe Prentice's Rule, decentration, and induced prism.
o   calculate induced prism and necessary decentration.

KEY POINTS

o   Distance between the pupil centers of both eyes is termed the *patient pupillary distance* (PD).
o   Distance between the centers of the right and left eye wires of the frame is the frame PD.
o   If the two centers do not coincide, prism is induced.
o   Prentice's Rule: (Induced prism, in PD or $^\Delta$) = (Lens power, in D) x (Optical center [OC] displacement, in cm).
o   Induced prism may be produced by calculating the amount of OC decentration.
o   The direction of the prism is always notated using the prism base.
o   In a plus lens, the base is displaced in the same direction as the OC.
o   In a minus lens, the base is displaced in the opposite direction as the OC.
o   Prisms oriented in the same direction are subtracted to obtain resultant prism.
o   Prisms oriented in the opposite direction are added to obtain resultant prism.
o   Optical labs typically split the prism between the two spectacle lenses.

DECENTRATION AND INDUCED PRISM

When prescription spectacle lenses are ordered, the optical shop measures the pupillary distance (PD)—the distance in mm between the pupil centers of both eyes—of the patient. This is termed the *patient PD* or *interpupillary distance* (IPD). In addition, the distance in mm between the centers of the right and left eye wires of the frame is also measured. This is termed the *frame PD* (Figure 25-1).

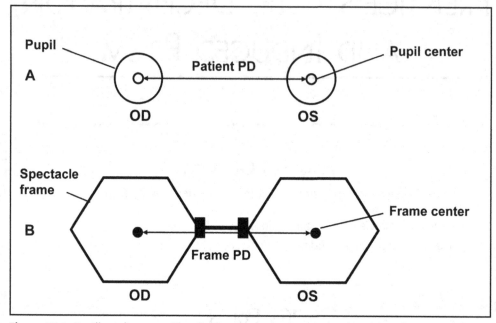

Figure 25-1. Pupillary distances. The distance between the center of each pupil is termed the patient pupillary distance, or patient PD (A). The distance between the center of OD and OS of the spectacle frame is termed the frame PD (B).

After the optical laboratory generates the prescription in a spectacle lens blank, the finished lens must be cut in such a way that 1) it properly fits into the spectacle frame, and 2) the optical center (OC) of the lens coincides with the center of the spectacle frame and the pupil center (Figure 25-2). This process of properly aligning the OCs of the lenses with the centers of the right and left eye wires of the spectacle frame and pupil centers of each eye is termed *decentration*. A proper decentration is accomplished by placing the finished lens on a template and moving it around to ensure that the lens OC is in the center of the eye wire of the spectacle frame and pupil. Accurate patient and frame PD measurements are required for this process.

A properly decentered pair of spectacle lenses will not only fit appropriately, but the patient's PD and frame PD will be the same so that the pupil and lens OCs coincide in each eye (Figure 25-2A). If the decentration is not properly accomplished, the two centers will not coincide in one or both lenses, resulting in unnecessary prism (called *induced prism*) (Figure 25-2B).

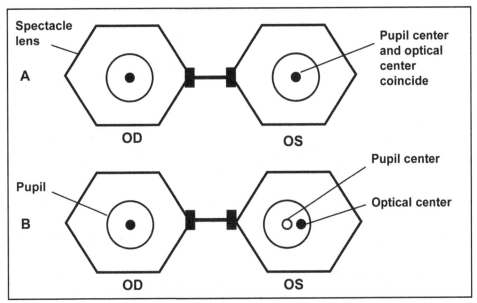

Figure 25-2. Fit of spectacle lenses. In properly fitting spectacle lenses, the pupil center of each eye and optical center of each spectacle lens coincide (A). When the two centers do not coincide, induced prism is produced, resulting in discomfort (B).

Unnecessary induced prism is very uncomfortable and includes symptoms such as[1]:

o   dizziness

o   nausea

o   pulling sensation in the eye

o   diplopia

Prism is frequently prescribed in spectacle lenses to eliminate diplopia or to ease astheno-pia. In single-vision glasses for spherical refractive errors, such prism is frequently produced as induced prism by using Prentice's Rule.

PRENTICE'S RULE

Prismatic effects are produced when looking through any part of a spectacle lens other than its OC. Conversely, prism may be intentionally induced (eg, for eliminating diplopia) by decentering the OC so that it does not coincide with the pupil center. The amount of induced prism (in prism diopters, abbreviated as PD or Δ) depends upon the power (in D) of the spectacle lens and the decentration, or OC displacement, (in cm) of the OC from the pupil center. (See Chapter 14 for details of prisms.)

Prentice's Rule relates these properties:

$$\text{Induced prism}_{(PD \text{ or } \Delta)} = \text{Lens power}_{(D)} \times \text{OC displacement}_{(cm)}$$

Where:

Induced prism =	measured in prism diopters (PD or Δ)
Lens power =	measured in diopters (as D)
OC displacement (decentration)	
=	measured in cm

Prentice's Rule may also be rearranged to determine the other variables: lens power or the OC displacement:

$$\text{Lens Power}_{(D)} = \frac{\text{Induced prism}_{(PD \text{ or } \Delta)}}{\text{OC displacement}_{(cm)}}$$

$$\text{OC Displacement}_{(cm)} = \frac{\text{Induced prism}_{(PD \text{ or } \Delta)}}{\text{Lens power}_{(D)}}$$

Prism is typically included in spectacle lenses for eliminating diplopia, and may be incorporated into the finished spectacle lens in two ways:

1. Generating the prism, along with the prescription, on the lens blank. Such lenses cannot be centered in a lensmeter.

2. Producing induced prism by calculating the amount of OC decentration using Prentice's Rule. Such lenses can be centered in a lensmeter. Therefore, prism should be checked after marking the OC on both spectacle lenses and comparing the frame PD to the patient PD.

As described in Chapter 14, the power of prisms is measured in PD or Δ. In ophthalmic usage, the direction of the prism is always notated using the prism base (Table 25-1).

Table 25-1	
Prism Base Orientation	**Notation**
Down (inferior)	Base down (BD)
Up (superior)	Base up (BU)
Nasally (medial)	Base in (BI)
Temporally (lateral)	Base out (BO)
Compound prism may also be present, and combines UP or DOWN with IN or OUT.	

The prism base orientation in induced prism depends on whether the lens is a plus or minus lens (Figures 25-3 and 25-4):

o   In a plus lens, the base is displaced in the same direction as the OC. If the OC is displaced UP, the prism is BU.

o   In a minus lens, the base is displaced in the opposite direction as the OC. If the OC is displaced UP, the prism is BD.

So far, we have dealt with prism present in only one eye. But what if prism is present in both eyes? The total, or resultant, prism in both eyes may be obtained by applying the following rule (Figures 25-5 through 25-8):

o   Prisms oriented in the same direction are subtracted to obtain resultant prism.

o   Prisms oriented in the opposite direction are added to obtain resultant prism.

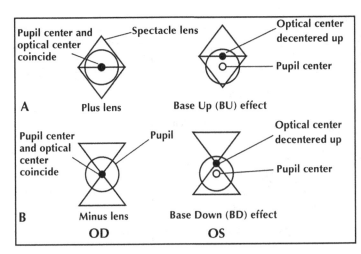

Figure 25-3. Decentration of spectacle lenses. In a plus lens, the optical center (OC) is displaced in the same direction as the prism base (A); whereas in a minus lens, the OC is displaced in the opposite direction as the prism base (B).

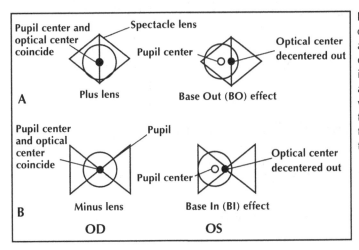

Figure 25-4. Decentration of spectacle lenses. In a plus lens, the optical center (OC) is displaced in the same direction as the prism base (A); whereas in a minus lens, the OC is displaced in the opposite direction as the prism base (B).

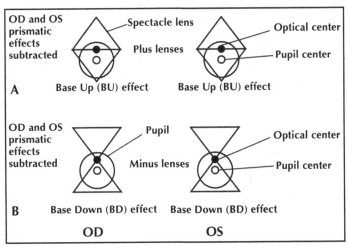

Figure 25-5. OD and OS prisms oriented in the same direction are subtracted, whether the lenses are plus (A) or minus (B) lenses.

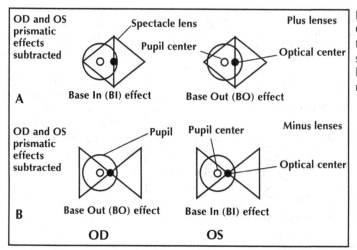

Figure 25-6. OD and OS prisms oriented in the same direction are subtracted, whether the lenses are plus (A) or minus (B) lenses.

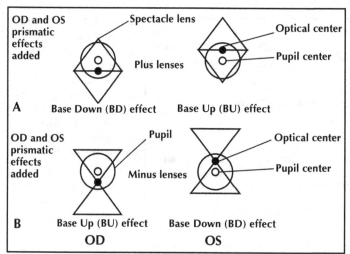

Figure 25-7. OD and OS prisms oriented in the opposite direction are added, whether the lenses are plus (A) or minus (B) lenses.

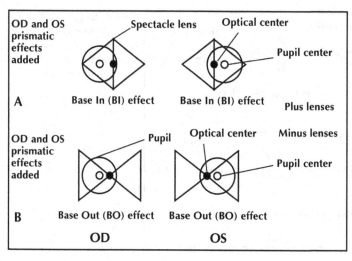

Figure 25-8. OD and OS prisms oriented in the opposite direction are added, whether the lenses are plus (A) or minus (B) lenses.

Example 1

Calculate the missing variable.

Lens Type and Power (D)	OC Displacement (cm)	Prism ($^\Delta$)	Direction of Base
OD: +5.00 sphere	?	1.5	BI

$$\text{OC displacement}_{(cm)} = \frac{\text{Induced prism}_{(\Delta \text{ or PD})}}{\text{Lens power}_{(D)}}$$

$$= \frac{1.5}{5}$$

$$= 0.3 \text{ cm}$$

$$= 3 \text{ mm}$$

Since it is a plus lens, the OC is displaced 3 mm in the same direction as the prism base (ie, nasally).

Example 2

Calculate the missing variable.

Lens Type and Power (D)	OC Displacement (cm)	Prism ($^\Delta$)	Direction of Base
OS: −4.00 sphere	?	0.8	BI

$$\text{OC displacement}_{(cm)} = \frac{\text{Induced prism}_{(\Delta \text{ or PD})}}{\text{Lens power}_{(D)}}$$

$$= \frac{0.8}{4}$$

$$= 0.2 \text{ cm}$$

$$= 2 \text{ mm}$$

Since it is a minus lens, the OC is displaced in the opposite direction as the prism base (ie, temporally).

Example 3

Calculate the missing variables.

Lens Type and Power (D)	OC Displacement (cm)	Prism ($^\Delta$)	Direction of Base
OS: −6.00	4 mm temporally	?	?

$$\text{Induced prism}_{(\Delta \text{ or PD})} = (\text{Lens power}_{(D)})\,(\text{OC displacement}_{(cm)})$$

$$= (6)\,(0.4)$$

$$= 2.4^\Delta$$

Since it is a minus lens, the prism base is in the opposite direction as the displaced OC (ie, base in).

Example 4

Calculate the missing variables.

Lens Type and Power (D)	OC Displacement (cm)	Prism ($^\Delta$)	Direction of Base
OD: +2.00	5 mm temporally	?	?

$$\text{Induced prism}_{(\Delta \text{ or PD})} = (\text{Lens power}_{(D)})(\text{OC displacement}_{(cm)})$$
$$= (2)(0.5)$$
$$= 1^\Delta$$

Since it is a plus lens, the prism base is in the same direction as the displaced OC (ie, base out).

Example 5

Calculate the missing variable.

Lens Type and Power (D)	OC Displacement (cm)	Prism ($^\Delta$)	Direction of Base
OD: ?	5 mm temporally	5.0	BI

$$\text{Lens power}_{(D)} = \frac{\text{Induced prism}_{(\Delta \text{ or PD})}}{\text{OC displacement}_{(cm)}}$$
$$= \frac{5}{0.5}$$
$$= 10 \text{ D}$$

Since the prism base (BI) is opposite to the OC displacement (temporally), the lens is a minus lens (ie, −10 D).

Example 6

Calculate the missing variable.

Lens Type and Power (D)	OC Displacement (cm)	Prism ($^\Delta$)	Direction of Base
OS: ?	3 mm nasally	1.5	BO

$$\text{Lens power}_{(D)} = \frac{\text{Induced prism}_{(\Delta \text{ or PD})}}{\text{OC displacement}_{(cm)}}$$
$$= \frac{1.5}{0.3}$$
$$= 5 \text{ D}$$

Since the prism base (BO) is opposite to the OC displacement (nasally), the lens is a minus lens (ie, −5 D).

Optical labs use the resultant concept, described above, to split the prism between the two lenses, thus enhancing the cosmetic effect of the two spectacle lenses. For example:

Prism Ordered	Prism Split by Optical Lab
OD: 6^Δ BO OS: —	OD: 3^Δ BO OS: 3^Δ BO
OD: 2^Δ BD OS: —	OD: 1^Δ BD OS: 1^Δ BU
OD: 6^Δ BO OS: 2^Δ BD	OD: 3^Δ BO 1^Δ BU OS: 3^Δ BO 1^Δ BD

Example 7

Calculate the total (resultant) prism given the following parameters:

$$OD: 5^\Delta \text{ BO}$$
$$OS: 4^\Delta \text{ BO}$$

Prisms in opposite directions are added.

Resultant = 9^Δ BO

Example 8

Calculate the total (resultant) prism given the following parameters:

$$OD: 4^\Delta \text{ BD}$$
$$OS: 3^\Delta \text{ BD}$$

Prisms in the same direction are subtracted.

Resultant = 4^Δ BD – 3^Δ BD

= 1^Δ BD OD

Reference

1. Shukla AV. Critical thinking protocols for ophthalmic medical personnel: refractometry. *J Ophthalmic Nursing & Technology.* 1999;18(1):24-28.

Review Questions

1.   A plus lens is:
    a.   two prisms attached base to base
    b.   two prisms attached apex to base
    c.   two prisms attached apex to apex
    d.   two prisms attached arbitrarily

2. What is the direction of induced prism in the Rx OD +2.00 sphere if the OC is displaced temporally?
    a.   BI
    b.   BU
    c.   BO
    d.   BD

3. What is the direction of induced prism if the patient looks above the OC with the Rx OD −6.00 sphere?
    a.   BD
    b.   BU
    c.   BO
    d.   BI

4. Induced prism can be calculated by Prentice's Rule, which can be mathematically expressed as:
    a. $Rx_{(D)} = $ Induced prism$_{(\Delta)} \times$ OC displacement$_{(mm)}$
    b.   OC displacement$_{(cm)} = \dfrac{\text{Induced prism}_{(\Delta)}}{Rx_{(D)}}$
    c.   OC displacement$_{(mm)} = \dfrac{Rx_{(D)}}{\text{Induced prism}_{(\Delta)}}$
    d.   Induced prism$_{(\Delta)} = \dfrac{\text{OC displacement}_{(mm)}}{Rx_{(D)}}$

5. How much will you need to decenter a lens, and in what direction, to produce the desired prismatic effect with the following parameters:

    Rx: OD +6.00 sphere

    Prescribed prism: 3^{Δ} BI
    a.   5 mm nasally
    b.   5 mm temporally
    c.   2 mm nasally
    d.   0.5 mm temporally

26

SPECTACLE LENSES

LEARNING OBJECTIVES

Upon completion of this chapter, the reader should be able to:

o   describe D_1 and D_2 surfaces, base curve, and power curves.
o   calculate radius of curvature and power of base curve.

KEY POINTS

o   The anterior curved surface of the spectacle lens provides plus power.
o   The posterior curved surface of the spectacle lens provides minus power.
o   The front surface (D_1) of the spectacle lens is the base curve.
o   The back surface (D_2) of the spectacle lens is the power curve.
o   The nominal power of a spectacle lens is $D_1 + D_2$.
o   The true power considers D_1, D_2, and refractive index.
o   The base curve of minus lenses is typically < +6 D.
o   The base curve of plus lenses is typically +6 D or greater.
o   The power curve gives the finished spectacle lens its characteristic thickness.
o   In minus lenses, the center of the lens is thinnest; in plus lenses, the center of the lens is thickest.
o   Slab-off reduces prismatic effects produced on looking down through the bifocal segment.

REFRACTION OF LIGHT THROUGH A SPECTACLE LENS

As described in Chapter 22, light refracted through a spectacle lens undergoes vergence changes in order to produce the desired state of corrected emmetropia. The anterior curved surface of the spectacle lens has plus power and imparts positive vergence (convergence) to light rays, whereas the posterior curved surface of the spectacle lens has minus power and imparts negative vergence (divergence) to light rays (Figure 26-1). The combination of plus and minus power together, along with refractive index (RI) of the lens material and its thickness, provide the prescribed lens power.

The RI of various spectacle lenses are listed below:

Glass:	Crown:	1.523
	Flint:	1.620
	Lantal:	1.900
Plastic:	High index:	1.500 to 1.670

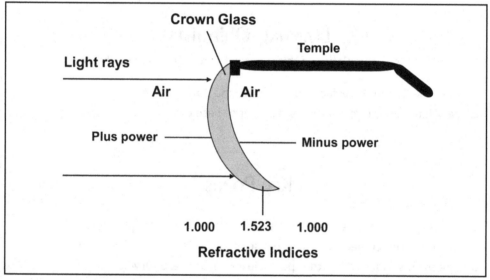

Figure 26-1. Light refraction through a spectacle lens. The anterior spectacle lens surface has plus power and converges light, whereas the posterior surface has minus power and diverges light. This combination, along with the refractive index of the lens material, produces the prescribed lens power.

THE CURVED REFRACTING SURFACES OF SPECTACLE LENSES

Optical lens manufacturers have established the following nomenclature for the curved refracting surfaces of spectacle lenses (Figure 26-2):
- Front surface (D_1) is the base curve of the lens, which imparts plus power. The base curve is set by manufacturers who produce *lens blanks* with various base curves.
- Back surface (D_2) is the power curve of the lens, which imparts minus power. The optical laboratory generates (ie, grinds) a specific curve to provide the power.

The *nominal power* of a spectacle lens is $D_1 + D_2$, which does not take RI into account. On the other hand, the true power takes all important variables (D_1, D_2, and RI) into account to determine the power of a lens.

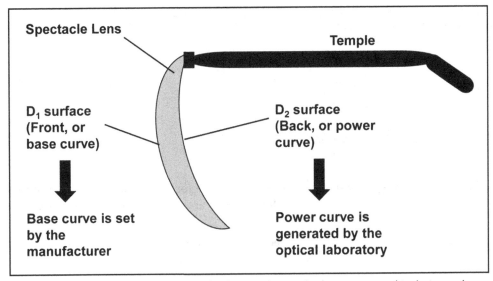

Figure 26-2. Spectacle lens in profile. The front surface is the base curve and is designated as D_1. The back surface is the power curve and is designated as D_2.

BASE CURVE

The base curve has a specific radius of curvature (r), which depends on the spectacle prescription, and may be measured using the black numbers of a *Geneva Lens Measure*:

o   Myopia: the base curve is generally < +6 D.

o   Hyperopia: the base curve is +6 D or greater.

Manufacturers produce lens blanks with a variety of base curves that can be used to generate the power curve.

Cheap nonprescription sunglasses are mass produced with a base curve of +4 D, which often causes distortions,[1] whereas good quality nonprescription sunglasses have a base curve of +6 D, which reduces or eliminates distortions.

POWER CURVE

The power curve has a specific r that depends on the spectacle prescription, and may be measured using the red numbers of a Geneva Lens Measure. The power curve is different for myopes and hyperopes, and gives the finished spectacle lens its characteristic thickness:

o   Myopia: a minus lens is its thinnest at the center.

o   Hyperopia: a plus lens is thickest at the center.

GENERATING THE POWER CURVE

Chapter 22 describes how the RI is an important variable in determining the power of a curved surface. That concept is applied to the power curves (back or D_2 surface) of spectacle lenses. Optical laboratories have standardized procedures based on this concept in order to *generate prescribed power curves* on spectacle lens blanks.

As previously described (Chapter 22), the power of a curved surface can be expressed mathematically:

$$P_{(D)} = \frac{(n_2 - n_1)}{r_{(m)}}$$

Where:

P = refractive power (in D)
n_1 = RI of air
n_2 = RI used to standardize lab tools
r = radius of curvature (in m) of lens curve

The formula can be rearranged to consider r in mm for ease of calculations. Since there are 1000 mm in a m, the numerator and denominator are multiplied by 1000 and the formula becomes:

$$P_{(D)} = \frac{1000\,(n_2 - n_1)}{1000\,r_{(m)}} = \frac{1000\,(n_2 - n_1)}{r_{(mm)}}$$

When optical laboratories were first established, the RI of lab tools (n_2) used to grind the power curve was standardized at 1.530. The formula now becomes:

$$P_{(D)} = \frac{1000\,(n_2 - n_1)}{r_{(mm)}}$$

$$P_{(D)} = \frac{1000\,(1.530 - 1.000)}{r_{(mm)}}$$

$$P_{(D)} = \frac{1000\,(0.530)}{r_{(mm)}}$$

$$P_{(D)} = \frac{530}{r_{(mm)}}$$

$$r_{(mm)} = \frac{530}{P_{(D)}}$$

Next, optical laboratories manufactured metal blocks, termed *tools*, with a top surface of a specific r using the formula above. The r varied in 0.25 D steps to generate prescribed powers in spectacle lenses. This is the reason that spectacle prescriptions are notated in 0.25 D increments, and powers specified in ⅛ D (eg, +2.375 D) will be rounded off to the closest lower 0.25 D (eg, +2.25 D) when the power curve is generated in the spectacle lens blank.

SLAB-OFF

In a spectacle lens with 2 D to 2.5 D of anisometropia, prismatic effects, as defined by Prentice's Rule, are created on looking down through the bifocal segment. Such prismatic effects induce vertical phorias, which may cause significant discomfort to the patient when looking through the bifocal segment. In such cases, optical laboratories use *slab-off* to eliminate the troubling prismatic effects.

Ophthalmic medical personnel (OMP) must be vigilant after completing refractometry and notify the ophthalmologist when significant anisometropia is present and slab-off should be considered. Additionally, prismatic effects must be suspected when a patient reports great discomfort when using the bifocal segment, and slab-off may be considered to alleviate the symptoms.

A prismatic effect is produced when gaze is directed from the optical center (OC) for distance toward the bifocal add segment, which has its own OC (Figure 26-3). In plus lenses, such gaze shift produces a BU effect, whereas in minus lenses, a BD effect is produced. The reading add segment, which is a plus lens, creates a BD effect. This, in turn, creates an *image jump* that may be very uncomfortable, especially in minus prescriptions.[2]

In a plus lens, the BU effect of the distance portion subtracts from the BD effect of the reading add segment, thus decreasing the image jump. In a minus lens, the BD effect of the distance portion is added to the BD effect of the reading add segment,[2] thus increasing the image jump.

The image jump in the two eyes will be similar if the vertical prismatic effect in the OD and OS is the same, and the patient might not complain of discomfort. However, if the vertical prismatic effects in the OD and OS are significantly different (produced by significant anisometropia), they will produce discomfort and an induced phoria in the eye with the greater prismatic effect.

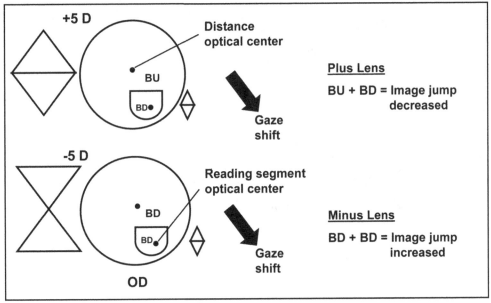

Figure 26-3. Image jump and slab-off, right spectacle lens. Prismatic effects are produced when gaze is directed from the distance optical center (OC) to the reading add segment OC (thick arrows). In a plus lens, the image jump is decreased (top), whereas in a minus lens, image jump is increased (bottom).

Prismatic effects can be calculated using Prentice's Rule, as shown below:

OD: +4.00 sphere
OS: +2.00 sphere   Add: +3.00 OU

Assume that the reading segment OC is 8 mm below distance OC.[2]

Vertical prism:	OD:	3.2$^\Delta$ BU
	OS:	1.6$^\Delta$ BU
	Total:	1.6$^\Delta$ BU (OD)

In this case, the 1.6$^\Delta$ BU OD will induce a hyperphoria because, when covered, the eye will drift upward, and when uncovered, the eye will turn downward, indicating a hyper deviation to the examiner. Note that the induced phoria (hyper) is opposite to the deviation that a BU prism would typically correct (hypo).

The undesirable prismatic effects may be eliminated by removing BD prism from the more minus or less plus lens. This is termed *slab-off* since the BD prism is "slabbed" off.

References

1. Stein HA, Stein RM, Freeman MI. *The Ophthalmic Assistant: A Text for Allied and Associated Ophthalmic Personnel*. 8th ed. Chicago, IL: Mosby; 2006.
2. Thall EH, Miller KM, Rosenthal P, Schechter RJ, Steinert RF, Beardsley TL. *Basic and Clinical Science Course, Section 3: Optics, Refraction, and Contact Lenses*. San Francisco, CA: American Academy of Ophthalmology; 2000.

Review Questions

1.   Minus power in all spectacle lenses is provided by:
     a.   the D_1 surface
     b.   the power curve
     c.   the cornea
     d.   the base curve

2.   The value of $D_1 + D_2$ is termed the:
     a.   base curve
     b.   true power
     c.   power curve
     d.   nominal power

3.   A lens blank base curve of +2 indicates that the glasses prescription:
     a.   is for a hyperope
     b.   decreases excess plus power
     c.   is for a presbyope
     d.   increases excess plus power

4.   Based on the nominal power of a lens, what is the power curve of a +2 D lens blank if the prescription is −4 D?
     a.   −6 D
     b.   +5 D
     c.   −5 D
     d.   +6 D

5. Compared to the image jump produced by OD: −3 D SPH, Add +3 D, the image jump produced by OD: +3 D SPH, Add +3 D will be:

    a.   less

    b.   the same

    c.   more

    d.   variable

27

CONTACT LENSES

LEARNING OBJECTIVES

Upon completion of this chapter, the reader should be able to:

o   describe D_1 and D_2 surfaces, base curve, and power curves.
o   calculate radius of curvature and power of base curve.

KEY POINTS

o   Front surface (D_1) is the power curve of the lens, which imparts plus power.
o   Back surface (D_2) is the base curve of the contact lens, and is set by manufacturers who make contact lenses with various base curves.
o   The flatter meridian is called "the K" and is used to determine the starting base curve.
o   The power (in diopters, or D) and the radius of curvature (r) (in mm) of the contact lens base curve may be calculated by dividing 337.5 by one or the other.
o   A 0.05 mm change in r is equivalent to a 0.25 D change in power.
o   Manifest refractometry (MR) in minus cylinder format is used because the flatter corneal axis is considered for fitting contact lenses.
o   The sphere portion of minus cylinder refractometry must be corrected for vertex distance.
o   Vertex distance is the distance between the spectacle plane and the corneal apex plane.
o   The power of plus lenses decreases with decreasing vertex.
o   The power of minus lenses increases with decreasing vertex.

KEY POINTS (CONTINUED)

o   Refractive errors greater than 4 D must be corrected for vertex.

o   In myopes, the contact lens sphere power will be less than the corresponding spectacles.

o   In hyperopes, the contact lens sphere power will be greater than the corresponding spectacles.

OPTICAL PARAMETERS OF CONTACT LENSES

(This chapter will be restricted to optical parameters of rigid gas-permeable [RGP] and soft contact lenses [SCL], and readers are encouraged to review other details of these contact lenses in standard textbooks on this subject.)

Contact lenses (RGP and SCL) have many uses (eg, correcting refractive errors, enhancing cosmetic appearance, masking the effects of disfiguring, using black occluder lenses for non-sighted eyes, helping corneal healing [bandage lenses], treating corneal conditions such as keratoconus and corneal irregularities, and occlusion therapy for amblyopia). Contact lenses do not affect image size as much as glasses do, and are well suited for monocular aphakia.[1,2]

The two optical parameters considered for RGP and SCL are corneal curvatures and contact lens power for correcting refractive error.

(As noted above, there are many other variables and considerations for deciding on RGP versus SCL, and readers are encouraged to review those details in standard textbooks on this subject.)

Corneal curvatures, which determine the base curve of contact lenses, may be measured using an ophthalmometer (Keratometer), or may be obtained from simulated keratometry (SIM-K) values included in computed corneal topography (CCT).

Contact lens powers for correcting refractive errors are obtained from manifest refractometry (MR) in minus cylinder format because the flatter corneal axis is considered for fitting contact lenses.

THE CURVED REFRACTING SURFACES OF CONTACT LENSES

Optical lens manufacturers have established the following nomenclature for the curved refracting surfaces of contact lenses (Figure 27-1):

o   Front surface (D_1) is the power curve of the lens, which provides plus power. The contact lens laboratory generates (ie, grinds) a specific curve to provide the power.

o   Back surface (D_2) is the base curve of the contact lens, and is set by manufacturers who make contact lenses with various base curves. Manufacturers notate the base curve in radius of curvature (r) in mm.

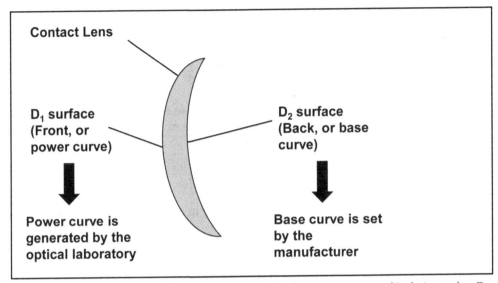

Figure 27-1. Contact lens in profile. The front surface is the power curve and is designated as D_1. The back surface is the base curve and is designated as D_2.

CONTACT LENS BASE CURVE

The first optical parameter to be considered for RGP and SCL is the *contact lens base curve*, which is based on measurements of corneal curvatures.

Since the back surface (D_2 or base curve) of a contact lens rests on the cornea, it must conform to corneal curvatures to ensure the best fit and comfort. The most common process is to measure the power of the cornea in diopters (D), and then convert it to r in mm.

The power of the cornea may be manually measured in two meridians mutually at 90 degrees by an ophthalmometer (Keratometer), which is calibrated to a refractive index (RI) of 1.3375. If the two meridians have equal powers, the cornea is spherical, whereas if the two meridians have different powers (maximum and minimum), the cornea is astigmatic. Astigmatic corneas may be classified based on the orientation of their steep axis:

- o Steep axis at 90 degrees = with-the-rule (W/R) corneal astigmatism
- o Steep axis at 180 degrees = against-the-rule (A/R) corneal astigmatism

Keratometry readings (also termed "K-readings" or "Ks") are typically notated in D by the contact lens fitter (eg, 43.00 @ 160 / 44.00 @ 70).

The flatter meridian is called *the K*, and is used to determine the starting base curve of a contact lens (eg, 44.50 @ 160 / 45.50 @ 70; the K = 44.50 D).

The K is further amended to derive the starting base curve for contact lenses. The procedures for doing so are different for RGP and SCL, and readers are encouraged to review those procedures in standard textbooks on contact lenses.

However, manufacturers typically notate the base curve of contact lens in r in mm [$r_{(mm)}$]. D may be converted to $r_{(mm)}$ by applying the concept of power of a curved surface (see Chapter 22), as was described for spectacle lenses (see Chapter 26):

$$P_{(D)} = \frac{(n_2 - n_1)}{r_{(m)}}$$

Where:

    P = refractive power (in D)

    n_1 = RI of air

    n_2 = RI used to standardize lab tools for contact lenses

    r = radius of curvature (in m)

Since the r of contact lenses is specified in m, the formula can be rearranged to consider r in mm for ease of calculations. Since there are 1000 mm in a m, the numerator and denominator are multiplied by 1000, and the formula becomes:

$$P_{(D)} = \frac{1000\,(n_2 - n_1)}{1000\,r_{(m)}} = \frac{1000\,(n_2 - n_1)}{r_{(mm)}}$$

The Keratometer was calibrated with a standardized RI of 1.3375 (note that the RI of tears is 1.336). The formula now becomes:

$$P_{(D)} = \frac{1000\,(n_2 - n_1)}{r_{(mm)}}$$

$$P_{(D)} = \frac{1000\,(1.3375 - 1.000)}{r_{(mm)}}$$

$$P_{(D)} = \frac{1000\,(0.3375)}{r_{(mm)}}$$

$$P_{(D)} = \frac{337.5}{r_{(mm)}}$$

$$r_{(mm)} = \frac{337.5}{P_{(D)}}$$

Thus, the power (in D) and the r (in mm) of the contact lens base curve may each be calculated by dividing 337.5 by one or the other.

Example 1

What is the base curve for a SCL with the following parameters:

        K-reading: 43.00 @ 180 / 44.00 @ 90

        The K: 43 D

  Starting base curve: 43 − 5 =   38 D*

  Radius of curvature: $r_{(mm)}$ = $\dfrac{337.5}{P_{(D)}}$

                      $r_{(mm)}$ = $\dfrac{337.5}{38}$

                      $r_{(mm)}$ = 8.8 mm

Thus, a SCL of 8.8 mm r and the proper lens power may be considered for fitting.

Readers are encouraged to consult standard textbooks on contact lenses to review procedures for altering the K to derive the starting base curve of contact lenses. These procedures are different for RGP and SCL.

Example 2

What is the power (in D) of a base curve with the following parameter:

        Base curve: 8.4 mm

Power: $P_{(D)}$ = $\dfrac{337.5}{r_{(mm)}}$

$P_{(D)}$ = $\dfrac{337.5}{8.4}$

$P_{(D)}$ =   40.17 D

Rounded off: $P_{(D)}$ =   40 D

Thus, the power of a base curve with an 8.4 mm r is 40 D.

Once inserted, the contact lens base curve may be further altered based on objective and subjective findings during the fitting session. Generally, a 0.05 mm change in r is equivalent to a 0.25 D change in power (1 D change = 0.2 mm change). Specific criteria are used to alter the starting base curve based on the fitting session, and readers are encouraged to consult standard textbooks to review these criteria.

CONTACT LENS POWER

The second optical parameter to be considered for RGP and SCL is the *contact lens power* for correcting the refractive error. Contact lens powers are obtained from MR in minus cylinder format because the flatter corneal axis is considered for fitting contact lenses. If refractometry is performed in plus cylinder, that measurement must be transposed to minus cylinder. As described in Chapter 24, the cylinder measured during refractometry represents the total astigmatism with components from the crystalline lens and cornea. Therefore, even though minus cylinder is used in contact lens fitting, because the lens is fit on the flatter (or minus cylinder) meridian, it is not entirely correct to assume that all of the minus cylinder is due to corneal astigmatism. However, this notion is widespread!

EXAMPLE 3

Refractometry result: −3.50 +0.50 x 80

Convert to minus cylinder format: −3.00 −0.50 x 170

VERTEX CORRECTION FOR CONTACT LENS POWER

Once the refractometry result is obtained in minus cylinder, the sphere portion of that measurement must be corrected for *vertex distance*, which is the distance between the spectacle plane and the corneal apex plane. Vertex distances are generally 11 to 13 mm, and may be accurately measured using a *Distometer*:

o   The patient is asked to wear the spectacles as they are normally worn.

o   The Distometer has two arms, one of which is placed on the closed upper eyelid.

o   A piston device is gently pushed (no squeezing), which places the other arm on the D_2 surface of the spectacle lens.

o   The vertex distance in mm is read on the scale.

o   The Distometer is calibrated so that 0.5 mm is added to account for typical upper eyelid thickness.

As described in Chapter 8, the power of any lens will change as it is brought closer to the cornea from the spectacle plane (ie, as the vertex distance decreases). All lenses lose plus power with decreasing vertex distance and, conversely, gain minus power with increasing vertex distance. Because of this, the following optical effects will occur with decreasing vertex:

o   The power of plus lenses decreases.

o   The power of minus lenses increases.

Up to refractive errors of 4 D, the changes in powers of plus and minus lenses due to decreasing vertex distance are insignificant, so no vertex correction is required. Refractive errors greater than 4 D must be corrected for vertex. The greater the refractive error, the greater the vertex corrected power. The following scheme should be noted for refractive errors greater than 4 D:

o   In myopes, the contact lens sphere power will be less than the corresponding spectacles.

o   In hyperopes, contact lens sphere power will be greater than the corresponding spectacles.

If a patient with a refractive error significantly greater than 4 D is given the same sphere power in a contact lens as in the corresponding spectacles, the patient will be blurred.

The following procedure may be used for completing vertex correction:

o   Obtain refractive error in minus cylinder and vertex distance.

o   Calculate the focal length $[f_{(mm)}]$ of the sphere (see Chapter 10).

o   To increase the power of a plus lens, subtract the vertex (in mm) from the $f_{(mm)}$.

o   To decrease the power of a minus lens, add the vertex (in mm) to the $f_{(mm)}$.

o   Use the newly determined $f_{(mm)}$ to calculate the power (D).

o   Round off to the closest lower 0.25 D.

o   This is the refractive error in minus cylinder that has been vertex corrected.

Example 4

Correct the following refractive error for fitting contact lenses, assuming a vertex of 12 mm:

$$+10.00 -2.00 \times 160$$

Calculate the focal length $[f_{(mm)}]$ of the sphere	=	+10 D
	=	100 mm
Plus lens: subtract the vertex (in mm) from $f_{(mm)}$	=	100 − 12
	=	88 mm
New $f_{(mm)}$ for calculating the power (D)	=	11.36 D
Round off to the closest lower 0.25 D	=	+11.25 D

A +10.00 −2.00 x 160 refractive error corrected for 12 mm vertex is +11.25 −2.00 x 160.

Example 5

Correct the following refractive error for fitting contact lenses, assuming a vertex of 12 mm:

$$-10.00 -2.00 \times 160$$

Calculate $f_{(mm)}$ of the sphere	=	−10 D
	=	100 mm
Minus lens: add the vertex (in mm) to $f_{(mm)}$	=	100 + 12
	=	112 mm
New $f_{(mm)}$ for calculating the power (D)	=	−8.9 D
Round off to the closest lower 0.25 D	=	−8.75 D

A −10.00 −2.00 x 160 refractive error corrected for 12 mm vertex is −8.75 −2.00 x 160.

Example 6

Correct the following refractive error for fitting contact lenses, assuming a vertex of 12 mm:

$$+8.00\ +2.00 \times 70$$

Refractive error in minus cylinder	=	+10.00 –2.00 × 160
Calculate $f_{(mm)}$ of the sphere	=	+10 D
	=	100 mm
Plus lens: subtract the vertex (in mm) from $f_{(mm)}$	=	100 – 12
	=	88 mm
New $f_{(mm)}$ for calculating the power (D)	=	11.36 D
Round off to the closest lower 0.25 D	=	+11.25 D

A +8.00 +2.00 × 70 refractive error corrected for 12 mm vertex is +11.25 –2.00 × 160.

Example 7

Correct the following refractive error for fitting contact lenses, assuming a vertex of 12 mm:

$$-12.00\ +2.00 \times 70$$

Refractive error in minus cylinder	=	+10.00 –2.00 × 160
Calculate $f_{(mm)}$ of the sphere	=	–10 D
	=	100 mm
Minus lens: add the vertex (in mm) to $f_{(mm)}$	=	100 + 12
	=	112 mm
New $f_{(mm)}$ for calculating the power (D)	=	–8.9 D
Round off to the closest lower 0.25 D	=	–8.75 D

A –12.00 +2.00 × 70 refractive error corrected for 12 mm vertex is –8.75 –2.00 × 160.

CONTACT LENS WORKUP

Standard textbooks should be consulted to review procedures for determining whether a patient is a candidate for RGP or SCL. The protocols described above for optical parameters (base curves and vertex correction of refractive errors) for contact lenses may be used in conjunction with other information obtained from reviewing standard textbooks.

REFERENCES

1. Stein HA, Stein RM, Freeman MI. *The Ophthalmic Assistant: A Text for Allied and Associated Ophthalmic Personnel.* 8th ed. Chicago, IL: Mosby; 2006.
2. Thall EH, Miller KM, Rosenthal P, Schechter RJ, Steinert RF, Beardsley TL. *Basic and Clinical Science Course, Section 3: Optics, Refraction, and Contact Lenses.* San Francisco, CA: American Academy of Ophthalmology; 2000.

Review Questions

1. The D_2 curved refractive surface in a contact lens is the:
    a.   power curve of a contact lens
    b.   base curve of a contact lens
    c.   optical center of a lens
    d.   base curve of a spectacle lens

2. Vertex refers to distance (mm) between the posterior surface of a spectacle lens and the:
    a.   anterior surface of the upper eyelid
    b.   anterior surface of the cornea
    c.   anterior surface of the lower eyelid
    d.   posterior surface of the cornea

3. Vertex measurements are important in refractive errors:
    a.   up to 4 D
    b.   of −4 D
    c.   greater than 4 D
    d.   of +4 D

4. As vertex distance is decreased, a spectacle Rx of +9.00 will most likely be:
    a.   +10.50
    b.   −9.25
    c.   +8.75
    d.   −7.50

5. As vertex distance is decreased, a spectacle Rx of −9.00 will most likely be:
    a.   +10.50
    b.   −9.25
    c.   +8.75
    d.   −7.50

Appendix:
Answers and Explanations
to Review Questions

Chapter 1

1. **a. 1300 mg/L**

   Since 1 L = 10 dL, using these units 130 mg/dL becomes 1300 mg/L.

2. **c. 0.05 dL**

   Since 1 dL = 100 mL, using these units 5 mL becomes 0.05 dL.

3. **a. 2 g**

   Since 4 x 500 mg = 2000 mg, and 1 g = 1000 mg, using these units 2000 mg becomes 2 g.

4. **a. 0.5 m**

   Since 1 m = 100 cm, using these units 50 cm becomes 0.5 m.

5. **b. the same**

   1000 mm = 1 m

Chapter 2

1. **a. 6**

   $$RI = \frac{3 \times 10^{10} \text{ cm per sec}}{\text{Speed of light in a medium}}$$

   $$RI = \frac{3 \times 10^{10}}{0.5 \times 10^{10}}$$

   $$RI = \frac{3}{0.5}$$

   $$RI = \frac{30}{5}$$

   $$RI = 6$$

2. **d. 0.6 x 10¹⁰ cm/sec**

   $$RI = \frac{3 \times 10^{10} \text{ cm per sec}}{\text{Speed of light in a medium}}$$

   $$\text{Speed of light in a medium} = \frac{3 \times 10^{10} \text{ cm per sec}}{RI}$$

   $$\text{Speed of light in a medium} = \frac{3 \times 10^{10}}{5}$$

   $$\text{Speed of light in a medium} = 0.6 \times 10^{10} \text{ cm/sec}$$

3.   **a. 0.27 m**

$$f_{(m)} = \frac{1}{P_{(D)}}$$

$$f_{(m)} = \frac{1}{3.75}$$

$$f_{(m)} = 0.27 \text{ m}$$

4.   **c. +5 D**

$$V = U + P$$
$$V = -(0.5) + (+5.5)$$
$$V = -0.5 + 5.5$$
$$V = +5 \text{ D}$$

5.   **d. 0.5**

$$\text{Magnification} = \frac{\text{Image size}}{\text{Object size}}$$

$$\text{Magnification} = \frac{3}{6}$$

$$\text{Magnification} = 0.5$$

6.   **b. 21 cm**

$$P = \frac{C}{D}$$

$$C = P \times D$$
$$C = 7 \times 3$$
$$C = 21 \text{ cm}$$

7.   **b. 0.5 m**

$$P = \frac{C}{D}$$

$$D = \frac{C}{P}$$

$$D = \frac{12}{24}$$

$$D = \frac{1}{2}$$

$$D = 0.5 \text{ m}$$

8.   **a. 0.4 D**

$$D = \frac{2}{r_{(m)}}$$

$$D = \frac{2}{5}$$

$$D = 0.4 \text{ D}$$

9.   **d. −0.5 D**

Half cylinder power: $\frac{1.00}{2} = -0.50$
Sphere power: 0
Spherical equivalent: (Sphere power) + (Half cylinder power)
Spherical equivalent: (0) + (−0.50)
Spherical equivalent: 0 − 0.50
Spherical equivalent: −0.5 D

10. **b. 48.2 D**

$$P_{(D)} = \frac{(n_2 - n_1)}{r_{(m)}}$$

$$P_{(D)} = \frac{(1.376 - 1.000)}{0.0078}$$

$$P_{(D)} = \frac{0.376}{0.0078}$$

$$P_{(D)} = 48.2 \text{ D}$$

11. **c. 53 mm**

$$P_{(D)} = \frac{530}{r_{(mm)}}$$

$$r_{(mm)} = \frac{530}{P_{(D)}}$$

$$r_{(mm)} = \frac{530}{10}$$

$$r_{(mm)} = 53 \text{ mm}$$

12. **c. 43.25 D**

$$P_{(D)} = \frac{337.5}{r_{(mm)}}$$

$$P_{(D)} = \frac{337.5}{7.8}$$

$$P_{(D)} = 43.25 \text{ D}$$

13. **b. 1 D**

$$\text{Age} >48: \text{amplitude} = 3 - [0.5 \frac{(\text{age} - 48)}{4}]$$

$$\text{amplitude} = 3 - [0.5 \frac{(64 - 48)}{4}]$$

$$\text{amplitude} = 3 - [0.5 \left(\frac{16}{4}\right)]$$

$$\text{amplitude} = 3 - [0.5 (4)]$$

$$\text{amplitude} = 3 - 2$$

$$\text{amplitude} = 1 \text{ D}$$

14. **a. 5^Δ**

$$\text{Induced prism}_{(\Delta \text{ or PD})} = \text{Lens power}_{(D)} \times \text{OC displacement}_{(cm)}$$

$$\text{Induced prism}_{(\Delta \text{ or PD})} = (5) \times (1)$$

$$\text{Induced prism}_{(\Delta \text{ or PD})} = 5$$

15. **b. 0.5 cm**

$$\text{Induced prism}_{(\Delta \text{ or PD})} = \text{Lens power}_{(D)} \times \text{OC displacement}_{(cm)}$$

$$\text{OC displacement}_{(cm)} = \frac{\text{Induced prism}_{(\Delta \text{ or PD})}}{\text{Lens power}_{(D)}}$$

$$\text{OC displacement}_{(cm)} = \frac{0.25}{0.5}$$

$$\text{OC displacement}_{(cm)} = 0.5 \text{ cm}$$

Chapter 3

1. **b. waves**

    Particles (**a.**) is incorrect since amplitude is a characteristic of waves.
    Fluorescence (**c.**) and polarization (**d.**) are incorrect since they are phenomena.

2. **d. $\lambda = \frac{c}{f}$**

    $\lambda = \frac{f}{c}$ (**a.**) is incorrect because $c = \lambda f$. Therefore, c must be a numerator to determine λ.
    $f = \frac{\lambda}{c}$ (**b.**) is incorrect because $c = \lambda f$. Therefore, c must be a numerator to determine f.
    $f = \lambda c$ (**c.**) is incorrect because $c = \lambda f$. Therefore, f can never be the product of λ and c.

3. **b. 400 to 700 nm**

4. **a. coherent and monochromatic**

    Monochromatic and out of phase (**b.**) is incorrect since laser light is always in phase.
    Coherent and diffuse (**c.**) is incorrect since laser light is never diffuse.
    Produced by spontaneous emission (**d.**) is incorrect since laser light is produced by stimulated emission.

5. **c. 180 degrees**

    Bothersome glare is produced by horizontal surfaces, which polarize light horizontally (ie, at 180 degrees).

6. **a. destructive interference**

    Waves not traveling together will be out of phase. Therefore, their interactions will produce destructive interference.
    Polarization (**b.**) is incorrect since it refers to the vibration direction.
    Emission (**c.**) is incorrect since it refers to the particle nature of light.
    Constructive interference (**d.**) is incorrect since this type of interference will require waves to be in phase.

7. **b. fluorescing light will have a longer wavelength**

    This is the basis of Einstein's theory of the phenomenon.
    Excitation and fluorescing lights will have the same wavelengths (**a.**) is incorrect since this will not observe Einstein's theory.
    Fluorescing and excitation lights will have the same color (**c.**) is incorrect since each color has a specific wavelength.
    Excitation light will have a longer wavelength (**d.**) is incorrect since this will not observe Einstein's theory.

Chapter 4

1. **b. 3×10^8 m/sec**

2. **d. slower**

$$\text{Speed of light} = \frac{3 \times 10^{10} \text{ cm per sec}}{RI} = \frac{3}{2} \times 10^{10} \text{ cm/sec} = 1.5 \times 10^{10} \text{ cm/sec}$$

$$\text{Speed of light} = \frac{3 \times 10^{10} \text{ cm per sec}}{RI} = \frac{3}{2.5} \times 10^{10} \text{ cm/sec} = 1.2 \times 10^{10} \text{ cm/sec}$$

3. **a. 1 x 10¹⁰ cm/sec**

$$\text{Speed of light} = \frac{3 \times 10^{10} \text{ cm per sec}}{RI} = \frac{3}{3} \times 10^{10} \text{ cm/sec} = 1 \times 10^{10} \text{ cm/sec}$$

4. **b. 2**

$$RI = \frac{3 \times 10^8 \text{ m per sec}}{\text{Speed of light}} = \frac{3 \times 10^8 \text{ m per sec}}{1.5 \times 10^8 \text{ m per sec}} = \frac{3}{1.5} = 2$$

5. **a. 2**

$$\text{Speed of light in medium} = 50\% \text{ slowing} = \frac{3 \times 10^{10} \text{ cm per sec}}{2} = \frac{3}{2} \times 10^{10} \text{ cm/sec}$$
$$= 1.5 \times 10^{10} \text{ cm/sec}$$

$$RI = \frac{3 \times 10^{10} \text{ cm per sec}}{\text{Speed of light}} = \frac{3 \times 10^{10} \text{ cm per sec}}{1.5 \times 10^{10} \text{ cm per sec}} = \frac{3}{1.5} = 2$$

Chapter 5

1. **a. shallower**

Light emerging from the pool of water bends away from the normal, thus making the pool appear shallower.

Darker (**b.**) and lighter (**d.**) are incorrect since other factors play a role in the pool appearing darker or lighter.

Deeper (**c.**) is incorrect since light rays emerging from the pool will bend away from the normal.

2. **d. bend at the interface**

Based on Snell's law, all rays will bend when they enter a transparent medium at an angle.

Not bend at the interface (**a.**) is incorrect since it does not observe Snell's law.

Be reflected (**b.**) is incorrect since only some rays, not all, might be reflected.

Be stopped (**c.**) is incorrect since the medium is transparent.

3. **d. $n_1 = n_2 \dfrac{\sin r}{\sin i}$**

Since Snell's law states that $n_1 \sin i = n_2 \sin r$, n_1 may be determined by moving $\sin i$ to the other side as a denominator.

$n_2 = n_1 \dfrac{\sin r}{\sin i}$ (**a.**), $n_1 = n_2 \sin i \sin r$ (**b.**), and $n_2 = n_1 \sin i \sin r$ (**c.**) are incorrect since rearranging Snell's law will not yield the answer choices shown.

4. **a. RI of the two media**

In Snell's law, the quantities n_1 and n_2 are refractive indices (RI) of the two media.

Reflection at the interface (**b.**) is incorrect since this phenomenon is not included in Snell's law.

The normal (**c.**) is incorrect since this is an imaginary line drawn at 90 degrees to the interface between two transparent media.

Sunlight (**d.**) is incorrect since it has nothing to do with Snell's law.

5. **c. bend toward the normal**

According to Snell's law, light traveling at an angle from a medium of lesser RI into a medium of greater RI will bend toward the normal.

Bend away from the normal (**a.**) is incorrect since it applies to light traveling at an angle from a medium of greater RI into a medium of lesser RI.

Continue without refraction along the normal (**b.**) is incorrect since it does not observe Snell's law.

Be reflected (**d.**) is incorrect since only some light rays, not all, will be reflected.

CHAPTER 6

1. **d. i_c will not apply**

Critical angle (i_c) only applies when light travels from a medium of greater refractive index (RI) into a medium of lesser RI, and does not apply when light travels from air into the eye.

The i_c can be calculated (**a.**) is incorrect since critical angle does not apply.

$r > i$ (**b.**) is incorrect since $r < i$ when light travels from the air into the eye.

All light will be reflected (**c.**) is incorrect since only some light, not all, is reflected.

2. **c. 1×10^8 m/sec**

$$\text{Speed of light} = \frac{3 \times 10^8 \text{ m per sec}}{\text{RI}} = \frac{3}{3} \times 10^8 \text{ m/sec} = 1 \times 10^8 \text{ m/sec}$$

3. **b. 0.5**

$$n_1 \sin i_c = n_2 \sin r$$
$$\sin i_c = \frac{n_2 \sin r}{n_1}$$
Since $\sin r = 1.0$,
$$\sin i_c = \frac{n_2}{n_1} = \frac{1}{2} = 0.5$$

4. **c. $r > 30$ degrees**

Since light travels from a medium of greater RI (2.000) into a medium of lesser RI (1.000), the refracted ray will bend away from the normal. Since the angle of incidence (i) is 30 degrees, the angle of refraction (r) will be greater than 30 degrees.

$r < 30$ degrees (**a.**) is incorrect since this condition applies when light travels from a medium of lesser RI into a medium of greater RI.

$i < 30$ degrees (**b.**) and $i > 30$ degrees (**d.**) are incorrect since the angle of incidence is stated as 30 degrees.

5. **a. $r < 30$ degrees**

Since light travels from a medium of lesser RI (1.000) into a medium of greater RI (2.000), the refracted ray will bend toward the normal. Since the i is 30 degrees, the r will be less than 30 degrees.

$i < 30$ degrees (**b.**) and $i > 30$ degrees (**d.**) are incorrect since the i is stated as 30 degrees.

$r > 30$ degrees (**c.**) is incorrect since this condition applies when light travels from a medium of greater RI into a medium of lesser RI.

Chapter 7

1. **d. there is no refraction**

    In total internal reflection (TIR), all light is reflected back into the first medium, and none is refracted into the second medium.

    The refracted ray bends toward the normal (**a.**) and the refracted ray bends away from the normal (**c.**) are incorrect since there is no refraction.

    Light goes from air into a gemstone (**b.**) is incorrect since TIR applies when light goes from a gemstone into the air.

2. **b. rays will be totally internally reflected**

    TIR applies since the angle of incidence (i; 50 degrees) exceeds the critical angle (i_c; 40 degrees) when light attempts to leave a medium of greater refractive index (RI; 1.523) into a medium of lesser RI (1.376).

    Refracted rays will bend away from the normal (**a.**), refracted rays will graze the interface between the media (**c.**), and refracted rays will bend toward the normal (**d.**) are incorrect since they apply to rays that are refracted, not totally internally reflected.

3. **a. from the angle structures toward the outside of the eye**

    TIR applies to this case, and all light from the angle structures is reflected back into the anterior chamber.

    From air into a fiber optic cable (**b.**), from air into a diamond (**c.**), and to the angle structures from the outside the eye (**d.**) do not apply since, in these answer choices, light travels from a medium of lower RI into a medium of greater RI.

4. **c. will not display TIR**

    Diamonds display TIR when numerous faces are cut on the crystal, thus creating the conditions of TIR. The orientations of crystal faces in uncut diamonds do not meet the conditions for TIR.

    Has dozens of crystal faces (**a.**) is incorrect since this number of faces have to be artificially cut.

    Has lots of fire (**b.**) is incorrect since the fire is created when faces are cut on the diamond to create conditions for TIR.

    May be expensive (**d.**) is incorrect since the true value of a diamond as a gemstone is redeemed when faces are cut on the diamond.

5. **b. a corneal cone**

    In keratoconus (corneal cone), the angle of incidence (i) may no longer exceed the critical angle (i_c), thus it does not meet the conditions of TIR. As a result, angle structures may be visible.

    Against the rule astigmatism (**a.**) is incorrect since TIR does not require astigmatism.

    Hypoglobus (**c.**) is incorrect since a globe displaced inferiorly will still meet the conditions of TIR.

    Microcornea (**d.**) is incorrect since conditions of TIR also apply to a smaller cornea.

Chapter 8

1. **a. plus lenses magnify images and display against motion of the image, whereas minus lenses reduce image size and display with motion of the image**

     These are the characteristics of plus and minus lenses.

     Plus lenses are thicker at the periphery (**b.**) is incorrect since plus lenses are thicker in the middle.

     Plus lenses reduce image size and display against motion of the image, whereas minus lenses magnify images and display with motion of the image (**c.**) is incorrect since the image size characteristics are incorrect.

     Minus lenses are thicker in the middle (**d.**) is incorrect since minus lenses are thicker at the periphery.

2. **b. have the same power in all meridians**

     This is the main characteristic of spherical lenses.

     Have different powers along various meridians (**a.**) is incorrect since this is the characteristic of spherocylindrical lenses.

     Only converge light (**c.**) and only diverge light (**d.**) are incorrect since plus and minus lenses can be spherical lenses.

3. **c. forms a line focus**

     This is the main characteristic of cylindrical lenses.

     Forms 30 degrees to the axis (**a.**) and forms 45 degrees to the axis (**b.**) are incorrect since the information presented in these choices is incomplete.

     Does not form (**d.**) is incorrect since an image forms as a line focus.

4. **b. –2.00 +2.00 x 90**

     The transposed form (PL –2.00 x 180) has plano power along the 180 axis, indicating that only one axis (90) has excess plus power (ie, myopia). Since one axis (180) does not require correction, whereas the other axis (90) is myopic, the type of astigmatism is simple myopic astigmatism.

     –2.00 +1.00 x 180 (**a.**) is incorrect since the transposed form (–1.00 –1.00 x 90) indicates that axis 90 is myopic. Since both axes are myopic, this is an example of compound myopic astigmatism.

     +2.00 –1.00 x 90 (**c.**) is incorrect since the transposed form (+1.00 +1.00 x 180) indicates that axis 180 is hyperopic. Since both axes are hyperopic, this is an example of compound hyperopic astigmatism.

     +2.00 +1.00 x 180 (**d.**) is incorrect since the transposed form (+3.00 –1.00 x 90) indicates that axis 90 is hyperopic. Since both axes are hyperopic, this is an example of compound hyperopic astigmatism.

5. **a. –2.00 +3.00 x 45**

     The transposed form (+1.00 –3.00 x 135) indicates that axis 135 is hyperopic. Since one axis (45) is myopic, whereas the other axis (135) is hyperopic, this prescription is an example of mixed astigmatism.

     +3.00 +2.00 x 135 (**b.**) is incorrect since the transposed form (+5.00 –2.00 x 45) indicates that axis 45 is also hyperopic. Since both axes are hyperopic, this prescription is an example of compound hyperopic astigmatism.

     –2.00 –3.00 x 45 (**c.**) is incorrect since the transposed form (–5.00 +3.00 x 135) indicates that axis 135 is also myopic. Since both axes are myopic, this prescription is an example of compound myopic astigmatism.

+3.00 +3.00 x 135 (**d.**) is incorrect since the transposed form (+6.00 –3.00 x 45) indicates that axis 45 is also hyperopic. Since both axes are hyperopic, this prescription is an example of compound hyperopic astigmatism.

CHAPTER 9

1.   **d. Law of Reflection**

Angle of incidence (i) = angle of reflection (r).

Snell's law (**a.**) is incorrect since it states $n_1 \sin i = n_2 \sin r$.

Refractive index (RI) (**b.**) is incorrect since it is $\dfrac{\text{Speed of light in a vacuum}}{\text{Speed of light in a medium}}$.

Total internal reflection (TIR) (**c.**) is incorrect since this applies to refraction.

2.   **a. reverse the direction of light travel**

All mirrors do this.

Provide plus power (**b.**) is incorrect since this is a characteristic of concave mirrors only.

Provide no power (**c.**) is incorrect since this is a characteristic of plane mirrors only.

Provide minus power (**d.**) is incorrect since this is a characteristic of convex mirrors only.

3.   **b. minus lenses**

Minus lenses and convex mirrors diverge light and provide minus power.

Plus lenses (**a.**) is incorrect since these lenses converge light and provide plus power.

No lenses (**c.**) is incorrect since mirrors may be compared to lenses.

Plano lenses (**d.**) is incorrect since convex mirrors have power, whereas plano lenses do not.

4.   **a. plus lenses**

Plus lenses and concave mirrors converge light and provide plus power.

Minus lenses (**b.**) is incorrect since these lenses diverge light and provide minus power.

No lenses (**c.**) is incorrect since mirrors may be compared to lenses.

Plano lenses (**d.**) is incorrect since concave mirrors have power, whereas plano lenses do not.

5.   **a. retinoscopy, gonioscopy, and slit lamp**

All of these procedures use instruments with mirrors.

Keratometry, trial lenses, and retinoscopy (**b.**) is incorrect since trial lenses do not have mirrors.

Computed corneal topography, retinoscopy, and Ishihara (**c.**) is incorrect since Ishihara color testing does not require mirrors.

Retinoscopy, gonioscopy, and stereo (**d.**) is incorrect since stereo testing does not require mirrors.

Chapter 10

1. **d. parallel light rays converge**

   This is the definition of focal point and focal length of a plus lens.

   Total internal reflection (TIR) occurs (**a.**) is incorrect since the focal point of a lens requires refraction.

   Parallel light rays appear to diverge from (**b.**) is incorrect since this is the definition for minus lenses.

   The Law of Reflection is observed (**c.**) is incorrect since the focal point of a lens requires refraction.

2. **b. parallel light rays appear to diverge from**

   This is the definition of focal point and focal length of a minus lens.

   TIR occurs (**a.**) is incorrect since the focal point of a lens requires refraction.

   The Law of Reflection is observed (**c.**) is incorrect since the focal point of a lens requires refraction.

   Parallel light rays converge (**d.**) is incorrect since this is the definition for plus lenses.

3. **a.** $f_{(cm)} = \frac{100}{P_{(D)}}$

   $f_{(m)} = \frac{100}{P_{(D)}}$ (**b.**) is incorrect since using $f_{(m)}$ requires the numerator to be 1.

   $P_{(D)} = \frac{100}{f_{(mm)}}$ (**c.**) is incorrect since using $f_{(mm)}$ requires the numerator to be 1000.

   $P_{(D)} = \frac{10}{f_{(cm)}}$ (**d.**) is incorrect since using $f_{(cm)}$ requires the numerator to be 100.

4. **b. 3.33 D**

   $$P_{(D)} = \frac{1000}{f_{(mm)}} = \frac{1000}{300} = \frac{10}{3} = 3.33$$

5. **c. 0.4 m**

   $$f_{(m)} = \frac{1}{P_{(D)}} = \frac{1}{2.5} = 0.4 \text{ m}$$

   $$f_{(cm)} = \frac{100}{P_{(D)}} = \frac{100}{2.5} = 40 \text{ cm}$$

Chapter 11

1. **c.** $V - P = U$

   The vergence equation is $U + P = V$, which may be rearranged ($V - P = U$) to determine the object vergence.

   $V + P = U$ (**a.**) is incorrect since $V - P = U$.

   $U - V = P$ (**b.**) is incorrect since $V - U = P$.

   $U - P = V$ (**d.**) is incorrect since $U + P = V$.

2. **c.** $D = \frac{1}{\text{distance}_{(m)}}$

   This is the formula for converting vergence to diopters (D), and vice versa.

3. **b. 0.02 D**

   Object distance (u) = 50 m

   Object vergence (U) = $\frac{1}{u_{(m)}} = \frac{1}{50} = 0.02$ D

4.   **a. +2.5 D**

    Object distance (u) = 500 mm

    Object vergence (U) = $\frac{1000}{u_{(mm)}}$ = $\frac{1000}{500}$ = $\frac{10}{5}$ = 2 D

    Image distance (v) = 2 m

    Image vergence (V) = $\frac{1}{v_{(m)}}$ = $\frac{1}{2}$ = 0.5 D

    Vergence equation: $U + P = V$
    Rearranging the equation to calculate power of a lens: $P = V - U$
    Minus sign added to U since the object is in minus space: $P = (V) - (-U)$
    $P = (0.5) - (-2)$
    $P = 0.5 + 2$
    $P = 2.5$ D

5.   **d. 33.3 cm in minus space**

    Object distance (u) = 400 cm

    Object vergence (U) = $\frac{100}{u_{(cm)}}$ = $\frac{100}{400}$ = $\frac{1}{4}$ = 0.25 D

    Power of lens (P) = −2.75 D
    Vergence equation: $U + P = V$
    Minus sign added to U since the object is in minus space: $V = -U + P$
    $V = (-0.25) + (-2.75)$
    $V = -0.25 - 2.75$
    $V = -3$ D
    Minus sign indicates that the image is located in minus space (before the lens).

    Image distance $[v_{(cm)}]$ = $\frac{100}{V}$ = $\frac{100}{3}$ = 33.3 cm

Chapter 12

1.   **d. 33.3 cm from the final lens and in its plus space**

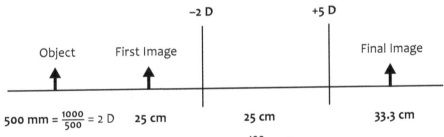

            First Lens
            $U + P = V$
          $(-2) + (-2) = V$
             $-2 - 2 = V$
              -4 D = V

        $f_{(cm)}$ = $\frac{100}{4}$ = 25 cm
        First image = 25 cm
         in minus space

            Second Lens
            $U + P = V$
         $(-2) + (+5) = V$
           $-2 + 5 = V$
            $+3$ D = V

       $f_{(cm)}$ = $\frac{100}{3}$ = 33.3 cm
      Final image = 33.3 cm
        in plus space

2. **b. at infinity in the plus space of the +1.00 lens**

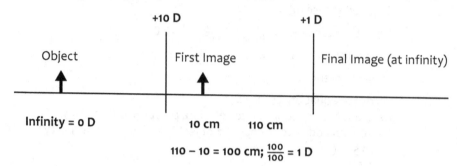

+10 D   +1 D

Object   First Image   Final Image (at infinity)

Infinity = 0 D   10 cm   110 cm

$$110 - 10 = 100 \text{ cm}; \frac{100}{100} = 1 \text{ D}$$

First Lens
$U + P = V$
$(-0) + (+10) = V$
$-0 + 10 = V$
$+10 \text{ D} = V$
$f_{(cm)} = \frac{100}{10} = 10 \text{ cm}$

First image = 10 cm
in plus space

Second Lens
$U + P = V$
$(-1) + (+1) = V$
$-1 + 1 = V$
$0 \text{ D} = V$
$f_{(cm)} = \frac{100}{0} = \text{infinity}$
(parallel rays)
Final image = at infinity
(parallel rays) in plus space

3. **a. 10 cm from the second lens and in its plus space**

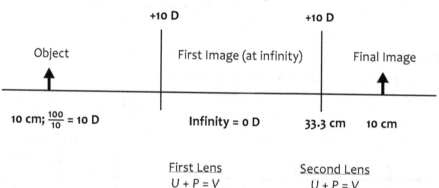

+10 D   +10 D

Object   First Image (at infinity)   Final Image

$10 \text{ cm}; \frac{100}{10} = 10 \text{ D}$ Infinity = 0 D   33.3 cm   10 cm

First Lens
$U + P = V$
$(-10) + (+10) = V$
$-10 + 10 = V$
$0 \text{ D} = V$
$f_{(cm)} = \frac{100}{0} = \text{infinity}$
(parallel rays)
First image = at infinity
(parallel rays) in plus space

Second Lens
$U + P = V$
$(-0) + (+10) = V$
$-0 + 10 = V$
$+10 \text{ D} = V$
$f_{(cm)} = \frac{100}{10} = 10 \text{ cm}$

Final image = 10 cm
in plus space

4. **d. 50 cm from the minus lens and in its minus space**

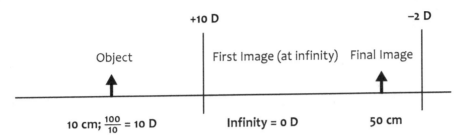

+10 D   −2 D

Object   First Image (at infinity)   Final Image

10 cm; $\frac{100}{10}$ = 10 D   Infinity = 0 D   50 cm

First Lens	Second Lens
$U + P = V$	$U + P = V$
$(-10) + (+10) = V$	$(-0) + (-2) = V$
$-10 + 10 = V$	$-0 - 2 = V$
$0\ D = V$	$-2\ D = V$
$f_{(cm)} = \frac{100}{0}$ = infinity	$f_{(cm)} = \frac{100}{2}$ = 50 cm
(parallel rays)	Final image = 50 cm
First image = at infinity	in minus space,
(parallel rays) in plus space	indicated by V = −2

5. **b. 25 cm from the second lens and in its minus space**

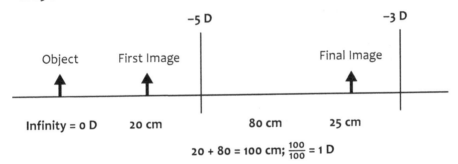

−5 D   −3 D

Object   First Image   Final Image

Infinity = 0 D   20 cm   80 cm   25 cm

20 + 80 = 100 cm; $\frac{100}{100}$ = 1 D

First Lens	Second Lens
$U + P = V$	$U + P = V$
$(-0) + (-5) = V$	$(-1) + (-3) = V$
$-0 - 5 = V$	$-1 - 3 = V$
$-5\ D = V$	$-4\ D = V$
$f_{(cm)} = \frac{100}{5}$ = 20 cm	$f_{(cm)} = \frac{100}{4}$ = 25 cm
First image = 20 cm	Final image = 25 cm
in minus space,	in minus space,
indicated by V = −5	indicated by V = −4

CHAPTER 13

1. **a. 1**

   Object distance (u): 1 m

   Object vergence (U): $\frac{1}{1} = 1$ D

   Power of lens (P): + 2 D

   Vergence equation: $V = U + P$

   A minus sign is assigned to U since the object is in the minus space of the lens.

   Image vergence: $V = -U + P$

   $V = (-1) + (+2)$

   $V = -1 + 2$

   $V = +1$ D

   Image distance: $\frac{1}{1} = 1$ m

   Magnification: $\dfrac{\text{Image distance}}{\text{Object distance}} = \frac{1}{1} = 1$

   The image is the same size as the object.

2. **c. 0.25**

   Object distance (u): 2 m

   Object vergence (U): $\frac{1}{2} = 0.5$ D

   Power of lens (P): −1.5 D

   Vergence equation: $V = U + P$

   A minus sign is assigned to U since the object is in the minus space of the lens.

   Image vergence: $V = -U + P$

   $V = (-0.5) + (-1.5)$

   $V = -0.5 - 1.5$

   $V = -2$ D

   Image distance: $\frac{1}{2} = 0.5$ m

   Magnification: $\dfrac{\text{Image distance}}{\text{Object distance}} = \dfrac{0.5}{2} = 0.25$

   The image is ¼ the size of the object.

3. **b. 5**

   Object size: 2 cm

   Image size: 10 cm

   Magnification: $\dfrac{\text{Image size}}{\text{Object size}} = \dfrac{10}{2} = 5$

   The image will be 5 times the size of the object.

4. **c. 50 cm**

   Object size: 5 cm

   Magnification: 10x

   Magnification: $\dfrac{\text{Image size}}{\text{Object size}}$

   Rearranging the equation to determine image size:

   Image size = (Magnification) x (Object size) = 10 x 5 = 50 cm

   The image will be 50 cm tall.

5.   **d. 20 cm**

Image size: 10 cm

Magnification: 0.5x

Magnification: $\dfrac{\text{Image size}}{\text{Object size}}$

Rearranging the equation to determine object size:

Object size: $\dfrac{\text{Image size}}{\text{Magnification}} = \dfrac{10}{0.5} = \dfrac{100}{5} = 20$ cm

The object is 20 cm tall.

Chapter 14

1.   **d. 4 cm**

$P = 2^\Delta$

$D = 2$ m

$C = (P)(D)$

$C = (2)(2)$

$C = 4$ cm

2.   **a. 500 cm**

$P = 0.5^\Delta$

$D = 1$ km $= 1000$ m

$C = (P)(D)$

$C = (0.5)(1000)$

$C = 500$ cm

3.   **b. 1 m**

$P = 10^\Delta$

$C = 100$ mm $= \dfrac{100}{10} = 10$ cm

$D = \dfrac{C}{P}$

$D = \dfrac{10}{10} = 1$ m

4.   **b. 0.25$^\Delta$**

$C = 5$ mm $= 0.5$ cm

$D = 2$ m

$P = \dfrac{C}{D}$

$P = \dfrac{0.5}{2} = 0.25^\Delta$

5.   **d. 0.1$^\Delta$**

$C = 100$ cm

$D = 1$ km $= 1000$ m

$P = \dfrac{C}{D}$

$P = \dfrac{100}{1000} = 0.1^\Delta$

Chapter 15

1.   **b. (D)(r) = 2**

$D = \dfrac{2}{r}$

$(D)(r) = 2$

2. **d. r = 2f**

$$f = \frac{r}{2}$$
$$2f = r$$

3. **b. 3 D**

$$f = 33 \text{ cm}$$
$$f = \frac{33}{100} \text{ m} = 0.33 \text{ m}$$
$$D = \frac{1}{f_{(m)}}$$
$$D = \frac{1}{0.33}$$
$$D = 3 \text{ D}$$

4. **b. 8 D**

$$r = 250 \text{ mm}$$
$$r = \frac{250}{1000} = 0.25 \text{ m}$$
$$D = \frac{2}{0.25} = \frac{200}{25} = 8 \text{ D}$$

5. **a. 50 cm**

$$D = \frac{1}{f_{(m)}}$$
$$f_{(m)} = \frac{1}{D}$$
$$f_{(m)} = \frac{1}{2}$$
$$f = 0.5 \text{ m} = 50 \text{ cm}$$

CHAPTER 16

1. **b. have the same power in all meridians**

    Have different powers along various meridians (**a.**) is incorrect since that is a characteristic of spherocylindrical lenses.

    Only converge light (**c.**) is incorrect since that is a characteristic of plus lenses, both spherical and cylindrical.

    Only diverge light (**d.**) is incorrect since that is a characteristic of minus lenses, both spherical and cylindrical.

2. **c. used to increase plus vergence**

    Plus lenses increase plus vergence (and decrease minus vergence), and their images form in plus space.

    –2 D (**a.**) is incorrect since that is a minus lens.

    Used to increase minus vergence (**b.**) is incorrect since that is a use of minus lenses.

    +5 D (**d.**) is incorrect since its focal length is 20 cm ($\frac{100}{5}$ = 20 cm).

3. **a. –2 D**

    Minus lenses decrease plus vergence (and increase minus vergence), and their images form in minus space.

    Used to decrease minus vergence (**b.**) is incorrect since minus lenses increase minus vergence.

Used to increase plus vergence (**c.**) is incorrect since that is the characteristic of plus lenses.

+5 D (**d.**) is incorrect since its focal length is 0.2 m ($\frac{100}{5}$ = 20 cm = 0.2 m).

4.   **c. lenses that reduce image sizes**

Patients with excessive plus vergence are myopic, meaning refractive error is corrected using minus lenses. Reducing image size is an important characteristic of minus lenses.

Lenses that magnify images (**a.**) is incorrect since that is a characteristic of plus lenses.

PL Sph (**b.**) is incorrect since myopic patients need refractive correction.

A +5 D lens (**d.**) is incorrect since a myope using plus lenses will become even more myopic.

5.   **a. lenses that magnify images**

Patients with inadequate plus vergence are hyperopic, meaning refractive error is corrected using plus lenses. Magnifying image size is an important characteristic of plus lenses.

PL Sph (**b.**) is incorrect since hyperopic patients need refractive correction.

Lenses that reduce image sizes (**c.**) is incorrect since that is a characteristic of minus lenses.

A −5 D lens (**d.**) is incorrect since a hyperope using minus lenses will become even more hyperopic.

CHAPTER 17

1.   **b. 167**

Cylinder axis: 77

Cylinder power is 90 degrees away: 77 + 90 = 167

2.   **d. 180**

Cylinder power required at axis: 90

Cylinder should be oriented 90 degrees away: 90 + 90 = 180

3.   **a. −1 D**

The total cylindrical power of a combination of cylindrical lenses, held with their axes parallel, is the algebraic (not arithmetic) sum of each power:

Total cylinder power with axes parallel: (+ 1) + (−2) = + 1 − 2 = −1 D

4.   **c. 0.5 D**

The cylindrical lenses in any Jackson Cross-Cylinder (manual or on a refractor) are of opposite signs and oriented with their axes at 90 degrees to each other. Cylindrical lenses oriented in such a way will manifest both powers, and the total cylindrical power of a combination of such lenses is the arithmetic (not algebraic) sum of each power:

Total power of cylindrical lenses of opposite signs and held with their axes at 90 degrees to each other: (0.25) + (0.25) = 0.5 D

Similarly, Jackson Cross-Cylinders with powers of ±0.50 D, ±0.75 D, and ±1 D will have total cylindrical powers of, respectively, 1 D, 1.5 D, and 2 D.

5.   **c. +2 D**

(Please see explanation for Question 4, above, for details.)

Total power of cylindrical lenses of opposite signs and held with their axes at 90 degrees to each other: (+1) + (+1) = 1 + 1 = 2 D

Chapter 18

1.   **d. +4.50 –1.50 x 180**

Plus cylinder to minus cylinder:

Plus cylinder:	+3.00	+1.50	x	90
	sphere	cylinder		cylinder
		power		axis

Algebraically add the sphere and cylinder:	(+3) + (+1.50) = +4.50
New sphere power:	+4.50
Copy the full cylinder power:	1.50
Change the sign of the cylinder power:	–1.50
Change the axis by 90 (180 is the maximum):	(90 + 90 = 180)
The transposed Rx is:	

Minus cylinder: +4.50   –1.50   x   180

2.   **a. +8.00 –4.00 x 90**

Plus cylinder to minus cylinder:

Plus cylinder:	+4.00	+4.00	x	180
	sphere	cylinder		cylinder
		power		axis

Algebraically add the sphere and cylinder:	(+4) + (+4) = +8
New sphere power:	+8.00
Copy the full cylinder power:	4.00
Change the sign of the cylinder power:	–4.00
Change the axis by 90 (180 is the maximum):	(180 – 90 = 90)
The transposed Rx is:	

Minus cylinder: +8.00   –4.00   x   90

3.   **b. two refracting surfaces**

Spherocylindrical lenses are combinations of spherical and cylindrical lenses. Such lenses have two refracting surfaces of different powers, which together produce the refraction characteristic of a spherocylindrical lens.

One plano surface (a.) and one refracting surface (d.) are incorrect since these are characteristics of cylindrical lenses.

Two plano surfaces (c.) is incorrect since this is a characteristic of lenses with no power.

4.   **a. spherocylindrical lenses**

Compound astigmatism must be corrected along two meridians with different powers. A lens with different powers along two meridians is a spherocylindrical lens.

Spherical lenses (b.) is incorrect since these lenses have the same power in all meridians, and correct myopia and hyperopia.

Cylinder lenses alone (c.) is incorrect since such lenses correct simple astigmatism.

Plano lenses (d.) is incorrect since these lenses do not have any power.

5.   **d. mixed astigmatism**
Plus cylinder form: –2.00 +4.00 x 87
Minus cylinder form: +2.00 –4.00 x 177
Plus power is excessive along one axis, requiring a minus lens (–2.00 at axis 87), and inadequate 90 degrees away, requiring a plus lens at that axis (+2.00 at axis 177). Such variations in plus power of the eye are characteristic of mixed astigmatism. In lens correction for mixed astigmatism, the cylinder power is greater than the sphere power, and of opposite sign.
Compound hyperopic astigmatism (**a.**) is incorrect since the sphere powers in plus and minus cylinder forms should be plus.
Compound myopic astigmatism (**b.**) is incorrect since the sphere powers in plus and minus cylinder forms should be minus.
Simple astigmatism (**c.**) is incorrect since the sphere power in plus and minus cylinder forms should have plano power along one axis, and plus or minus power along the other axis.

Chapter 19

1.   **b. spherical lens**
It is a spherical lens because both axes have the same power (+2).
Cylindrical lens with axis at 90 (**a.**) is incorrect because the other axis (180) has power.
Cylindrical lens with axis at 180 (**c.**) is incorrect because the other axis (90) has power.
Spherocylindrical lens (**d.**) is incorrect because both axes have the same power.

2.   **c. cylindrical lens with axis at 180**
This is because only one axis has power, and axis 180 is plano.
Cylindrical lens with axis at 90 (**a.**) is incorrect because the power is at axis 90.
Spherical lens (**b.**) is incorrect because both axes do not have the same powers.
Spherocylindrical lens (**d.**) is incorrect because only one axis has power.

3.   **d. spherocylindrical lens**
It is a spherocylindrical lens because both axes have power, but of different amounts.
Cylindrical lens with axis at 90 (**a.**) and cylindrical lens with axis at 180 (**c.**) are incorrect because both axes have power.
Spherical lens (**b.**) is incorrect because both axes have different powers.

4.   **b. –3.00 –2.00 x 180**
This is because –5 + PL = –5 at axis 90, and –5 + 2 = –3 at axis 180.
+5.00 –2.00 x 90 (**a.**) is incorrect because axis 90 does not have +5 of power.
–5.00 +2.00 x 180 (**c.**) is incorrect because axis 180 does not have –5 of power.
+3.00 +2.00 x 90 (**d.**) is incorrect because axis 90 does not have +3 of power.

5.   **a.**

Transposing the lens powers indicates that axis 90 has −1 and axis 180 has
+2.

−1.00 +3.00 x 90
+2.00 −3.00 x 180
(b.), **(c.)**, and **(d.)** do not show those powers.

Chapter 20

1.   **b. +3.00**

Lens prescription: +4.00 −2.00 x 90

Half cylinder power: $\frac{-2.00}{2}$ = −1.00
Sphere power: +4.00
Spherical equivalent: (Sphere power) + (Half cylinder power)
(+4) + (−1.00)
+4 − 1.00
+3.00

2.   **c. +4.50**

Lens prescription: +4.00 +1.00 x 90

Half cylinder power: $\frac{1.00}{2}$ = +0.50
Sphere power: +4.00
Spherical equivalent: (Sphere power) + (Half cylinder power)
(+4) + (+0.50)
+4 + 0.50
+4.50

3.   **c. +0.25 D**

Lens prescription: PL +0.50 x 75

Half cylinder power: $\frac{0.50}{2}$ = +0.25
Sphere power: 0.00
Spherical equivalent: (Sphere power) + (Half cylinder power)
(0) + (+0.25)
0 + 0.25
+0.25

4.   **d. −2.00**

Lens prescription: −1.75 −0.50 x 55
Spherical equivalent: (Sphere power) + (Half cylinder power)

$(−1.75) + (\frac{-0.50}{2})$
(−1.75) + (−0.25)
−1.75 − 0.25
Spherical soft lens power: −2.00

5.   **a. −2.25**

−2.50 +0.50 x 100
Lens prescription: −2.50 +0.50 x 100
Convert to minus cylinder: −2.00 −0.50 x 10

Spherical equivalent: (Sphere power) + (Half cylinder power)

$(-2.00) + (\frac{-0.50}{2})$

$(-2.00) + (-0.25)$

$-2.00 - 0.25$

Spherical soft lens power: -2.25

Chapter 21

1.   **b. 5**

Tears, cornea, aqueous, lens, and vitreous.

2.   **d. air-tears; tears-anterior cornea; posterior cornea-aqueous**

Posterior cornea-anterior cornea; posterior lens-vitreous; tears-aqueous (**a.**), air-tears; anterior cornea-posterior cornea (**b.**), and tears-vitreous; anterior cornea-air; aqueous-vitreous; air-vitreous (**c.**) are not in correct anatomical sequences.

3   **a. emmetropia**

Simple astigmatism (**b.**), ametropia (**c.**), and compound astigmatism (**d.**) are all caused by inappropriate amounts of refraction.

4.   **c. schematic reduced eye**

Emmetropic eye (**a.**), refractive eye (**b.**), and ametropic eye (**d.**) are not terms used in this context.

5.   **c. 2.44 cm**

Gullstrand assigned a length of 24 mm, which is equal to 2.44 cm.

24 cm (**a.**) is approximately equal to 9.5 inches; 24 m (**b.**) is approximately equal 26.25 yards; and 2.44 mm (**d.**) is equal to 0.244 cm. Therefore, these choices are incorrect.

Chapter 22

1.   **c. radius of curvature**

Refractive index (**a.**), angle of incidence (**b.**), and angle of refraction (**d.**) are incorrect since they have been considered previously.

2.   **a. $n_2 = [P_{(D)}] [r_{(m)}] + n_1$**

Equations (**b.**), (**c.**), and (**d.**) are not rearranged correctly.

3.   **a. the power will decrease by half**

Since the denominator (r) is doubled from 1 m to 2 m, the resulting fraction will decrease by half.

4.   **d. it will decrease**

"Applanation" means to make plane, which increases the radius of curvature (r). Because of this, the denominator in the fraction will increase, thus decreasing the power of the cornea until it resumes its original shape. Therefore, choices (**a.**), (**b.**), and (**c.**) are incorrect.

5. **b. 2 D**

n_1 = air = 1.000

n_2 = 1.200

Diameter = 20 cm = 200 mm

r = radius of curvature = $\dfrac{\text{diameter}}{2}$ = $\dfrac{200}{2}$ = 100 mm

$P_{(D)} = \dfrac{1000\,(n_2 - n_1)}{r_{(mm)}}$

$P_{(D)} = \dfrac{1000\,(1.200 - 1.000)}{100}$

$P_{(D)} = \dfrac{1000\,(0.200)}{100}$

$P_{(D)} = \dfrac{200}{100}$

$P_{(D)} = 2\ D$

6. **a. the r will increase**

In the equation for the power of a curved surface, if P is reduced and ($n_2 - n_1$) is unchanged, then the value of $r_{(m)}$ must increase.

$P(D) = \dfrac{(n_2 - n_1)}{r_{(m)}}$

The r will decrease (**b.**) is incorrect since decreasing the r will increase the power.

The r will be unaffected (**c.**) is incorrect since changing power and keeping the refractive indices (RI) unchanged will mathematically affect the r.

The r should not be considered (**d.**) is incorrect since that variable is part of the equation.

7. **d. increase**

n_1 = air = 1.000

n_1 = aqueous = 1.336

n_2 = IOL = 1.890

IOL implanted: $P_{(D)} = \dfrac{1000\,(n_2 - n_1)}{r_{(m)}} = \dfrac{1000\,(1.890 - 1.336)}{r_{(m)}} = \dfrac{1000\,(0.554)}{r_{(m)}} = \dfrac{554}{r_{(m)}}$

IOL in air: $P_{(D)} = \dfrac{1000\,(n_2 - n_1)}{r_{(m)}} = \dfrac{1000\,(1.890 - 1.000)}{r_{(m)}} = \dfrac{1000\,(.89)}{r_{(m)}} = \dfrac{890}{r_{(m)}}$

With $r_{(m)}$ unchanged, the value of $\dfrac{890}{r}$ is greater than the value of $\dfrac{554}{r}$.

Remain unchanged (**a.**) and decrease (**b.**) are incorrect since changing n1 from 1.000 to 1.890 and keeping $r_{(m)}$ constant will increase the value of P. Fluctuate (**c.**) is incorrect since "fluctuate" does not apply.

CHAPTER 23

1. **d. contraction of the ciliary muscle**

Contraction of zonules (**a.**) is incorrect since zonules are not muscle fibers and do not contract.

Contraction of the anterior capsule (**b.**) is incorrect since the capsule does not contract.

Relaxation of the ciliary muscle (**c.**) is incorrect since relaxation of the ciliary muscle stretches the zonules, thus making the lens thinner and allowing it to focus distant light rays.

2.   **b. increase in anterior lens capsule convexity**
        Increase in zonule length (**a.**) and relaxation of the ciliary muscle (**c.**) are incorrect since these occur when the lens focuses at distance.
        Increase in lens density (**d.**) is incorrect since this is an abnormal physiological condition seen in diabetes mellitus.

3.   **b. +19 D to +33 D**

4.   **d. plus lens**
        PL lens (**a.**) is incorrect since such a lens has no power.
        Minus lens (**b.**) is incorrect since minus lenses stimulate accommodation.
        Prism (**c.**) is incorrect since prisms are used to establish fusion.

5.   **a. +76 D**
        (+14) + (+62) = +76 D
        +62 D (**b.**) is incorrect since +62 D is the total power of a non-accommodating eye (+43 D from the air-tear-cornea-aqueous complex, and +19 D from the non-accommodating lens).
        +33 D (**c.**) is incorrect since +33 D is the maximum power of a lens at maximum accommodation (+14 D and +19 D).
        +19 D (**d.**) is incorrect since that is the total accommodative amplitude of a lens.

Chapter 24

1.   **b. ametropia**
        Myopia (**a.**) is incorrect since the question does not state whether the plus power is excessive.
        Hyperopia (**c.**) is incorrect since the question does not state whether the plus power is inadequate.
        Emmetropia (**d.**) is incorrect since this is the condition of an appropriate amount of plus power.

2.   **a. myopia**
        Decreasing the radius of curvature will increase the plus power.
        Ametropia (**b.**) is incorrect since the question states that the plus power changes a specific way.
        Hyperopia (**c.**) is incorrect since a decrease in the radius of curvature will increase the power.
        Emmetropia (**d.**) is incorrect since this condition, being of an appropriate amount of plus power, will no longer apply if the radius of curvature is changed.

3.   **c. hyperopia**
        Hyperopia requires more plus power, which is provided by accommodation.
        Myopia (**a.**) is incorrect since this condition already has excessive plus power, and providing more plus power by accommodating will increase the myopia.
        Ametropia (**b.**) is incorrect since hyperopia is already ametropia.
        Emmetropia (**d.**) is incorrect since this is the condition of an appropriate amount of plus power.

4.   **c. may be given +2.75 D**

Since + 2.00 D is the absolute hyperopia and +0.75 D is the facultative (manifest) hyperopia, the latter may (or may not) be given.

Absolute hyperopia (A): +2.00 (patient first reads 20/20)
Manifest hyperopia (M): +0.75 (patient continues to read 20/20)
Cycloplegic refractometry (CR): Information not provided

Type of Hyperopia	Definition	Spectacle Lens Correction
Latent	Corrected by accommodation	No plus lens needed (they will cause blurring)
Manifest (facultative)	Corrected by accommodation or by plus lenses	Plus lenses may be used but are not necessary
Absolute	Corrected by plus lenses only	Plus lenses necessary

Must be given +2.75 D (**a.**) is incorrect since the +0.75 may, or may not, be given.

Must be given +0.75 D (**b.**) is incorrect since +0.75 D is the facultative (manifest) hyperopia, whereas it is the absolute hyperopia (+2.00 D) that must be corrected.

May be given +0.75 D (**d.**) is incorrect since this power will not correct the absolute hyperopia.

5.   **c. may be given +1. 75 D**

This is the sum of absolute and manifest hyperopia.
Absolute hyperopia (A): +1.00 (patient first reads 20/20)
Manifest hyperopia (M): +0.75 (patient continues to read 20/20)
Absolute + Manifest (A + M): (+1.00) + (+0.75) = +1.75
Cycloplegic refractometry (CR): +3.50 D
Latent hyperopia (L):

$$L = CR - (A+M)$$
$$L = +3.50 - (+1.00 + 0.75)$$
$$L = +3.50 - (+1.75)$$
$$L = +3.50 - 1.75$$
$$L = +1.75$$

(see Table above)

Must be given +3.50 D (**a.**) and may be given +3.50 D (**d.**) are incorrect since those amounts also include +1.75 D of latent hyperopia, which must not be corrected.

Must be given +0.75 D (**b.**) is incorrect since +0.75 is the manifest hyperopia and may or may not be given.

6.   **b. 1.5 D of A/R preop lenticular astigmatism**

Preop manifest refractometry: +2.00 SPH
Postop manifest refractometry: −0.50 +1.50 x 87
Postoperatively, the patient has 1.5 D of W/R astigmatism corneal astigmatism,

which was masked by equal and opposite (1.5 D of A/R) astigmatism from the cataractous lens. When that lens was removed, the pre-existing corneal astigmatism was unmasked.

1.5 D of A/R postop corneal astigmatism (**a.**) is incorrect since the steeper axis is vertical.

0.5 D of W/R postop corneal astigmatism (**c.**) is incorrect since the measured cylinder is 1.5 D.

1.5 D of W/R preop lenticular astigmatism (**d.**) is incorrect since the 1.5 D of lenticular astigmatism has to be A/R in order to mask the 1.5 D of W/R corneal astigmatism.

CHAPTER 25

1. **a. two prisms attached base to base**

Two prisms attached apex to base (**b.**) is incorrect since that morphology is not seen.

Two prisms attached apex to apex (**c.**) is incorrect since that relates to minus lenses.

Two prisms attached arbitrarily (**d.**) is incorrect since that morphology is not seen.

2. **c. BO**

In a plus lens, the optical center (OC) displacement and prism base orientation are in the same direction. Here, it is temporal, or out.

BI (**a.**) is incorrect since that will occur if the OC is displaced nasally.

BU (**b.**) and BD (**d.**) are incorrect since the OC is displaced horizontally, not vertically.

3. **b. BU**

In a minus lens, the OC displacement and prism base orientation are in the opposite. Here, the OC is displaced down since the patient looks above it.

BD (**a.**) is incorrect since, for that to happen, the OC must move in the opposite direction (up) when the patient looks below it.

BO (**c.**) and BI (**d.**) are incorrect since the OC is displaced vertically, not horizontally.

4. **b. OC displacement$_{(cm)}$** $= \dfrac{\text{Induced prism}_{(\Delta)}}{Rx_{(D)}}$

5. **a. 5 mm nasally**

Lens Type and Power (D)	OC Displacement (cm)	Prism ($^\Delta$)	Direction of Base
OD: +6.00 sphere	?	3	BI

$$OC\ displacement_{(cm)} = \frac{\text{Induced prism}_{(\Delta\ or\ PD)}}{\text{Lens power}_{(D)}}$$
$$= \frac{3}{6}$$
$$= \frac{1}{2}$$
$$= 0.5\ cm$$
$$= 5\ mm$$

Since it is a plus lens, the OC is displaced 5 mm in the same direction as the prism base (ie, nasally).

CHAPTER 26

1. **b. the power curve**

    This is also the back (D_2) surface.

    The D_1 surface (**a.**) is incorrect since that is the base curve and always provides plus power.

    The cornea (**c.**) is incorrect since that is irrelevant information.

    The base curve (**d.**) is incorrect since it always provides plus power.

2. **d. nominal power**

3. **b. decreases excess plus power**

    Base curves less than +6 D are typically used for myopic prescriptions, which decrease the excess plus power that is characteristic of myopia.

    Is for a hyperope (**a.**) is incorrect since base curves for hyperopic prescriptions are +6 D or greater.

    Is for a presbyope (**c.**) is incorrect since that information is not provided.

    Increases excess plus power (**d.**) is incorrect since base curves less than +6 D are typically used for myopic prescriptions, which decrease the excess plus power that is characteristic of myopia.

4. **a. –6 D**

    $D_1 = +2$ D
    D_2 = power curve
    Nominal power = -4 D
    Nominal power = $D_1 + D_2$
    Rearranging equation to determine D_2:
    D_2 = (Nominal power) – (D_1)
    $ = (-4) - (+2)$
    $ = -4 - 2$
    $ = -6$ D

5. **a. less**

    The BU effect of the plus power distance correction will counteract the BD effect produced by the bifocal segment.

    The same (**b.**) is incorrect since the OD lens is minus, whereas the OS lens is plus.

    More (**c.**) is incorrect since BU effect of the plus power distance correction will counteract the BD effect produced by the bifocal segment.

    Variable (**d.**) is incorrect since the image jump effects are precise.

CHAPTER 27

1. **b. base curve of a contact lens**

    Power curve of a contact lens (**a.**) and base curve of a contact lens (**d.**) are incorrect since the question is about contact lenses.

    Optical center of a lens (**c.**) is incorrect since the optical center is measured on the D2 surface but marked on the D_1 surface of a spectacle lens.

2.   **b. anterior surface of the cornea**

Anterior surface of the upper eyelid (**a.**) is incorrect since vertex is measured from the cornea, and the measuring instrument includes 0.5 mm to allow for the thickness of a normal upper eyelid.

Anterior surface of the lower eyelid (**c.**) is incorrect since vertex parameters are measured from the upper eyelid.

Posterior surface of the cornea (**d.**) is incorrect since vertex involves the anterior surface of the cornea.

3.   **c. greater than 4 D**

Vertex distance is measured in all refractive errors greater than 4 D.

Up to 4 D (**a.**) is incorrect since up to 4 D of refractive error vertex distance does not make any difference.

Of −4 D (**b.**) and of +4 D (**d.**) are incorrect since vertex distance is an important variable in all refractive errors of 4 D and greater.

4.   **a. +10.50**

In hyperopia, greater than +4 D, the contact lens power should be more than the corresponding spectacle lens power.

+8.75 (**c.**) is incorrect for the reason stated above.

−9.25 (**b.**) and −7.50 (**d.**) are incorrect since these powers are for myopia.

5.   **d. −7.50**

In myopia, greater than −4 D, the contact lens power should be less than the corresponding spectacle lens power.

+10.50 (**a.**) and +8.75 (**c.**) are incorrect since these powers are for hyperopia.

−9.25 (**b.**) is incorrect since in myopia, the contact lens power should be less than the corresponding spectacle lens power.

Glossary

A

accommodative amplitude: the total change in the dioptric power of the crystalline lens.

accommodative effort: contraction of the ciliary muscle to initiate accommodation in normal phakic eyes; also occurs in normal aphakic and pseudophakic eyes, neither of which have an accommodative response.

accommodative esotropia: turning of the eyes toward the nose during accomodation, thus creating an esodeviation due to the synkinetic response (also termed the *synkinetic reflex*).

accommodative need: the dioptric equivalent of the distance at which a near object is customarily held; determined by calculating the inverse of the distance, in meters, of the near object.

accommodative range: the measurable range within which a near object appears in focus while looking through a reading add.

accommodative response: a change in the dioptric power of the crystalline lens in response to an accommodative effort.

against motion: in lenses, the motion of the image movement observed as a plus lens; in retinoscopy, the motion of the streak observed in an uncorrected myopic eye.

amblyopia: *ambly* = lazy; *opia* = vision; condition of unilateral or bilateral decrease in best-corrected vision, which cannot be ascribed to a structural defect in the eye.

ametropia: condition of the presence of a refractive error.

amplitude: the total spread or range of a feature, such as accommodation.

angle of incidence (*i*): the angle between incident light rays and the normal (an imaginary line drawn at 90 degrees to a surface) during refraction or reflection.

angle of refraction (*r*): the angle between refracted light rays and the normal (an imaginary line drawn at 90 degrees to a surface) during refraction.

angle structures: anatomical structures (trabecular meshwork and Canal of Schlemm) located in the periphery of the anterior chamber from where most of the aqueous humor exits the eye.

animals: rows of characters used to measure stereo acuity in seconds of arc.

aphakic: *a* = no; *phak* = lens; pertaining to the absence of a crystalline lens in the eye.

aqueous: *aqueous humor*, the liquid produced by the ciliary processes in the posterior chamber, which moves through the pupil into the anterior chamber, exiting the eye through the angle structures.

argon (Ar): element used as a lasing medium in lasers for treating retinal abnormalities.

astigmatic: *a* = no; *stigma* = point; denoting the absence of a point focus, which is seen in spherical spectacle and contact lenses, and spherical corneas and crystalline lenses, but not seen in cylindrical and spherocylindrical spectacle and contact lenses, or cylindrical and spherocylindrical corneas and crystalline lenses.

astigmatic ametropia: condition of the presence of a refractive error due to uncorrected astigmatism.

astigmatic image: denoting line images formed by cylindrical and spherocylindrical spectacle and contact lenses, and cylindrical and spherocylindrical corneas and crystalline lenses.

astigmatism: *a* = no; *stigma* = point; denoting a line image formed by cylindrical and spherocylindrical spectacle and contact lenses, and cylindrical and spherocylindrical corneas and crystalline lenses.

> *Regular astigmatism:* line image(s) correctable by lenses; includes simple myopic in which only one meridian is corrected by moving the line image from an anterior position to the fovea; simple hyperopic in which only one meridian is corrected by moving the line image from a posterior position to the fovea; compound myopic in which both meridia are corrected by moving the line images from anterior positions to the fovea; compound hyperopic in which both meridia are corrected by moving the line images from posterior positions to the fovea; and mixed in which one line image is moved from an anterior position to the fovea, whereas the other line image is moved from a posterior position to the fovea.
>
> *With-the-rule:* astigmatism in which the steeper meridian is vertical.
>
> *Against-the-rule:* astigmatism in which the steeper meridian is horizontal.
>
> *Total astigmatism:* sum of astigmatism of the cornea and the crystalline lens.
>
> *Irregular astigmatism:* line images not correctable by spectacle or soft contact lenses (SCL), but by rigid gas-permeable (RGP) contact lenses or surgery.

away from the normal: bending of refracted light rays when they pass from a medium of greater refractive index into a medium of lesser refractive index.

axial view: the most common view of corneal curvatures and powers displayed in computed corneal topography (CCT).

axis: the plane meridian, without refracting power, of a cylindrical lens.

B

back surface (D$_2$): in spectacle lenses, the posterior (power) surface, which is ground to the prescription specifics; in contact lenses, the posterior (base curve) surface, which rests on the cornea and, therefore, must have an appropriate curve.

balancing: in prescriptions, adding half of the available accommodative amplitude to the distance refractometry results to derive a balanced prescription in hyperopic children; in refractometry, adjusting the sphere power to make binocular images equally blurry to ensure that accommodation is not used for distance.

base curve: in contact lenses, the back (posterior, or D$_2$) surface, which rests on the cornea and must have an appropriate curve; in spectacle lenses, the front (anterior, or D$_1$) surface, which has a specific curve set by the manufacturer.

base out prism: prism oriented so that its base is toward the temple and the apex toward the nose, thus producing fusion in esotropia and esophoria.

blood glucose: concentration of glucose in blood, measured in milligrams per deciliter (mg/dL).

blue: along with violet, the shortest wavelength (greatest frequency) of visible light in the electromagnetic spectrum.

blue light: visible light of short wavelength (high frequency) used to excite fluorescein sodium, an orange ophthalmic dye.

brightness acuity test (BAT): used to quantify decrease in best corrected visual acuity in presence of progressively increasing bright light.

C

central (chief) ray: light rays along the principal axis of a lens, which are not refracted since they are incident at 90 degrees to the lens surface; clinically applied to measuring pinhole visual acuity.

central posterior curve: base curve of a contact lens.

ciliary muscle: intraocular sphincter muscle whose contraction initiates accommodative effort.

Circle of Least Confusion: in spherocylindrical lenses, the central point between the two line images produced by the two sphere powers in transposed prescriptions; dioptric value corresponds to the spherical equivalent.

circles within squares: sequence of 10 squares with four circles within each square that become progressively harder to distinguish and are used to quantify stereo vision in seconds of arc.

cobalt blue filter: located on biomicroscopes and some hand-held ophthalmic instruments, and used to excite yellow-orange fluorescein sodium dye. Resulting fluorescence is green and is used for applanation tonometry and evaluating the cornea and contact lenses.

cold laser: Nd:YAG laser used to destroy the central portion of a posterior capsule opacity using micro-explosions instead of heat.

compound astigmatism: regular astigmatism in which line images of both meridians do not form on the fovea, but either anteriorly (compound myopic astigmatism) or posteriorly (compound hyperopic astigmatism).

computed corneal topography (CCT): instrument with automated programs used to measure corneal power, radius of curvature, ectasia (abnormal stretching and bulging), and astigmatism.

concave mirror: reflecting surface that converges incident light rays.

concave-mirror effect: used to estimate hyperopia using a streak retinoscope by moving the collar vertically to produce a sharp (enhanced) streak. When this is achieved by moving the collar halfway, a maximum of +5 D of plus power is provided.

Conoid of Sturm: in spherocylindrical lenses, the distance between the two line images produced by the two sphere powers in transposed prescriptions.

constructive interference: positive interference produced by waveforms traveling in-phase.

contact lens base curve: the central portion of the back (posterior, or D_2) surface of a contact lens, which rests on the cornea and, therefore, must have an appropriate curve.

contact lens power: prescribed power for correcting a refractive error; generated on the front (D_1) surface of the lens.

convergence: in optics, positive vergence produced by light rays that converge after refraction or reflection.

convergence insufficiency: eye deviation in which divergence is greater at near than at distance.

convex mirror: reflecting surface that diverges incident light rays.

Copeland: a brand of streak retinoscope.

corneal alignment: device on a refractor to quantify vertex distance for refractometry by aligning a corneal profile with a reference line. If provided, the device is located lateral to the large wheel used to change sphere powers in 0.25 D increments.

corneal epithelium: anterior-most layer of a 5-layered normal cornea.

corneal irregularities: topographic irregularities on a cornea, resulting in irregular astigmatism.

corneal plane: an imaginary surface tangential to the greatest anterior position of a corneal profile.

cover testing: identification and measurement of a phoria or tropia by covering one eye at a time.

crests: highest point of a wave located 90 degrees above the wave baseline.

critical angle (i_c): angle of incidence at which the corresponding refracted ray grazes the interface between two media of different refractive indices, when light passes from a greater refractive index medium into a lesser refractive index medium.

crystalline lens: anatomic structure in a normal phakic eye that provides positive vergence (convergence, or plus power).

cycloplegic refractometry (CR): subjective measurement of a refractive error after producing cycloplegia of the ciliary muscle to rule out influence of accommodation.

cylinder axis: the orientation of the plane surface of cylindrical and spherocylindrical lenses that does not have any power.

cylinder power: power provided by the curved surface of cylindrical and spherocylindrical lenses, which is oriented at 90 degrees to the cylinder axis.

cylindrical lens: transparent refracting medium in which one surface is plane and has no refracting power, while the other surface is curved and has refracting power.

curved surface: one of two surfaces of a cylindrical lens providing all the power.

D

decentration: process used by optical labs to move the optical center of a spectacle lens and align it with the pupil center of the patient.

destructive interference: negative interference produced by waveforms traveling out-of-phase.

diabetes mellitus: abnormal condition resulting from nonsecretion of, or insensitivity to, insulin, and causing elevated levels of blood glucose.

diamonds: artificial gemstone produced by cutting numerous faces at appropriate angles in order to produce total internal reflection, which results in luster, and "fire."

diplopia: *diplo* = double; *opia* = vision; condition of double vision.

dispersion: separation of white light into its component colors after refraction through a prism or water droplets acting as prisms.

distometer: ophthalmic instrument for measuring the distance, in millimeters, between the closed upper eyelid and the back (posterior, or D_2) surface of a spectacle lens.

divergence: in optics, negative vergence produced by light rays that diverge after refraction or reflection.

duochrome: *duo* = two; *chrom* = color; red-green test commonly used in refractometry.

E

electromagnetic spectrum: measurable sequence of wavelengths, some of which are visible to the human eye, produced by the interplay of electrical and magnetic fields.

ellipses: oval-shaped geometric patterns whose radius varies from a maximum to a minimum value.

emmetropia: condition of the absence of a refractive error in an eye; also used when corrective lenses are introduced in front of the eye to correct a refractive error.

enhanced streak: a sharp streak produced during retinoscopy in a hyperopic meridian by moving a streak retinoscope collar vertically, thus providing the necessary plus power.

equation: a mathematical expression in which one or more variables are equal to other variable(s).

estimating hyperopia: a sharp streak may be produced during retinoscopy in a hyperopic meridian by moving a streak retinoscope collar vertically, thus providing the necessary plus power.

excimer: *exc* = excited; *imer* = dimer; laser used in photorefractive and phototherapeutic surgery (eg, PRK, LASIK, and LASEK).

excitation wavelength (blue): wavelength of light (eg, blue) that shines on a fluorescent substance (eg, fluorescein sodium) inducing it to produce light of a longer wavelength (eg, green).

excited-dimer: see *excimer.*

exophthalmometer: ophthalmic instrument used to quantify proptosis in one or both eyes.

extracapsular cataract extraction (ECCE): extraction (removal) of the material located inside the capsule of a cataractous crystalline lens by leaving most of the capsule intact. In ECCE by *expression*, the lens material is extracted by squeezing it through a large incision in the sclera. In ECCE by *phacoemulsification*, the lens material is first broken up into small pieces (emulsification) using sound waves produced by an instrument introduced into the eye through a small incision on the peripheral cornea, and the emulsified material is removed by aspiration.

eye exercises: fixating at a small object, approaching the eyes along the medial plane of the body (in an attempt to increase convergence and decrease the near point of convergence) in patients with convergence insufficiency.

F

far point: the farthest point that is in focus; generally the refractive error.

farsightedness: ability to see far away but not at near, a characteristic of hyperopia.

fiber optic cable: a coaxial set of transparent cables in which the material of the inner cable has a greater refractive index than the material of the outer cable, thus producing total internal reflection.

final image: the last image produced by a system of multiple lenses.

fire: in optics and gemology, refers to the great amounts of light escaping from inside a diamond through some crystal faces but not others, thus giving the impression of a fire.

fixation light: any small light used to direct the fixation of a patient.

flatter cornea: a cornea, typical of curvature hyperopia, whose radius of curvature is greater than normal and dioptric power is less than normal.

flatter meridian: the axis, in any refractive material, that has a radius of curvature greater than the steeper meridian and dioptric power less than the steeper meridian.

fluorescein angiogram: a record of fluorescence produced when fluorescein sodium is excited by blue light.

fluorescein sodium: orange-colored ophthalmic dye that emits green light when excited by blue light. May be given by an intravenous injection or orally.

fluorescence: an effect produced when fluorescent material is excited by light of a particular wavelength inducing the material to emit light of a longer wavelength.

fluorescent wavelength (green): color of emitted light when fluorescein sodium is excited by blue light.

fluorescing light: light of a specific wavelength emitted by a fluorescent material when excited by light of a shorter wavelength.

fly: a test of gross stereo vision.

focal length: in lens, distance at which an image forms in a plus lens, or appears to come from in a minus lens. In mirror, half the radius of curvature.

fogging: procedure used to ensure that excess minus, or inadequate plus, power is not introduced during refractometry.

frequency: number of waves that pass a point in unit time, typically one second.

Fresnel prisms: plastic prisms affixed on a spectacle lens to establish whether the measured
prism is adequate for the patient's need.

Fresnel searchlight: prisms of increasing apex angle used to refract light and produce a
powerful light beam, which is shined from lighthouses to assist naval vessels in navigating
treacherous waters off a coast.

front surface (D₁): the anterior surface of a corrective lens.

G

generating power curve: optical laboratory process to reshape the back surface of a spectacle lens blank in order to generate the prescribed dioptric power.

Geneva lens measure: optical instrument with a dial and prongs used to measure the front
and back curvature, in diopters, of spectacle lenses.

Goldmann applanation tonometer: conical biprism used to measure intraocular pressure by
applanating a standard portion of the cornea.

Goldmann lens: a mirrored contact lens held against an anesthetized cornea for gonioscopy.

Goldmann perimeter: bowl-shaped ophthalmic instrument used for manual plotting of monocular and binocular visual fields while the patient fixates on a target.

gonioscopy: process of viewing the angle and its structures.

green light: visible light in the electromagnetic spectrum whose wavelength is longer than
blue but shorter than yellow, orange, and red.

H

Herpes simplex: a DNA virus that causes characteristic dendritic lesions on the cornea.

hydroxylpropylmethylcellulose (Goniosol): viscous gel used to eliminate air and total internal
reflection during gonioscopy.

hyperopia (hypermetropia): condition of ametropia in which sharp images form posterior
to the fovea, thus indicating presence of inadequate positive vergence (plus power) and
requiring plus lenses for correction.

　　Axial: hyperopia caused by shorter-than-average globe length, measured from the pupil
center to the retina.

　　Curvature: hyperopia caused by greater-than-average radius of curvature of the cornea,
thus resulting in less-than-average power measured in diopters.

　　Absolute: component of hyperopia that requires correction by plus lenses.

　　Manifest (facultative): component of hyperopia that is corrected by accommodation or
plus lenses.

　　Latent: component of hyperopia that does not require correction.

　　Induced: hyperopia caused by excess minus (or inadequate plus) in corrective lenses.

hyperopic correction: plus lenses used to correct ametropia in which sharp images form
posterior to the fovea, thus indicating presence of inadequate positive vergence (plus
power).

hyperopic shifts: changes in the refractive status of the eye that decrease plus vergence (plus
power), thus moving sharp images from the fovea to a posterior location, and requiring
plus lenses for correction.

I

image distance: distance (in meters) of an image produced by a lens.

image jump: upward jump produced by the base-down effect of a reading add segment; corrected by using slab-off.

image size: dimension of an image produced by refraction or reflection of incident light rays.

image vergence: divergence or convergence of refracted rays (expressed in diopters), and obtained by the inverse (in meters) of the distance of an image from a lens.

incident light: incoming light rays toward a lens or mirror.

induced phoria: eye deviation induced by using unnecessary prism.

induced prism: prismatic effect induced by decentering the optical center of a spectacle lens away from the pupil center of an eye.

inferior cone: abnormal ectactic condition, a characteristic of keratoconus, in which increase in curvature of the cornea occurs inferior to the visual axis.

infrared (IR): portion of the invisible electromagnetic spectrum whose frequency is less than the red color of the visible spectrum.

in phase: wave propagation in which crests and troughs of all waves travel together.

interface: refracting surface present between two transparent media. The following interfaces are involved with refraction of incident light rays in a normal eye: air-tear; tear-anterior cornea; posterior cornea-aqueous; aqueous-anterior lens; posterior lens-vitreous.

interference: wave propagation in which crests and troughs of all waves either travel together (constructive interference) or not (destructive interference).

intraocular lens (IOL): artificial lens made from nonreactive substances and implanted in an eye with or without extracting the crystalline lens.

Anterior chamber IOL: implanted anterior to the iris.

Calculations: mathematical manipulations using axial length and keratometry measurements to calculate the optimal power (in diopters) of an IOL for implantation.

Posterior chamber IOL: implanted posterior to the iris.

intraocular pressure: pressure inside the eye dependant on production and outflow of aqueous humor.

K

keratoconus: abnormal condition in which the cornea develops a cone-shaped protrusion, causing ectasia, degeneration, and blurry vision.

Keratometer: trademarked name for an ophthalmometer, patented by Bausch & Lomb.

keratometry: measurement of the radius of curvature and/or dioptric power of a cornea.

Koeppe lens: one of many types of contact lenses used for gonioscopy.

krypton: element used as a lasing medium in lasers.

L

LASEK: acronym for laser sub-epithelial keratomileusis, a refractive surgery procedure used to reshape the cornea in order to alter its optics.

LASER (laser): acronym for Light Amplification by Stimulated Emission of Radiation.

LASIK: acronym for laser in situ keratomileusis, a refractive surgery procedure used to reshape the cornea in order to alter its optics.

Law of Reflection: in mirrors, angle of incidence is equal to the angle of reflection.

lens axis: the plane (uncurved), nonrefracting surface of a cylindrical lens.

lens blank: transparent medium of known base curve, with no power, used by optical laboratories to generate a finished spectacle lens with prescribed powers; used for single vision, bi- and tri-focal, and progressive addition lenses.

lens power: focusing power of lens measured in diopters.

lens vergence: divergence or convergence (expressed in diopters) imparted by a lens to incident rays, and obtained by the inverse (in meters) of the focal length of a lens.

lensometry: measurement of the power of a spectacle or contact lens.

light: visible portion (approximately 400 to 700 nm) of the electromagnetic spectrum.

light bending: refraction of light by a lens or prism by altering its path as it passes through the material.

line focus: longitudinal image formed by a cylindrical lens.

M

magnification: term used to denote both the magnification and reduction of an image produced by a refracting or reflecting medium.

manifest refractometry (MR): subjective measurement of a refractive error when the ciliary muscle is not temporarily paralyzed.

meniscus lens: a lens with two curves (bicurve), such as a spectacle and contact lens.

meridian: term used interchangeably with "axis."

metric: pertaining to meter, the measurement system using milli-, centi-, deci-, and kilo- as prefixes.

microexplosions: condition caused by Nd:YAG laser to destroy the central portion of a posterior capsule opacity around the visual axis.

minus cylinder form: system of denoting lens powers for correcting astigmatism using minus cylindrical lenses.

minus direction: more minus in minus lenses, or less plus in plus lenses.

minus lens: a refracting medium that provides negative vergence (divergence) and, thus, minus power.

minus power: negative vergence (divergence).

minus space: space before a lens through which light must pass to be incident on a refracting medium.

miosis: condition of pupil constriction.

mirror: a plane or curved reflecting medium with many uses: automobile, trucks, security, traffic, flashlights, bathroom, dressing, shaving, makeup, dentistry, microscopes, and ophthalmic instruments.

mixed astigmatism: ametropia in which one image forms anterior to the fovea and the other forms posterior to it.

monochromatic: *mono* = one; *chrom* = color; pertaining to one color.

monocular aphakia: condition of the absence of a crystalline lens in one eye.

multiple lens systems: an array of two or more lenses that alters the path of incident light.

muscle imbalances: abnormal function of the extraocular muscles involved with moving the eye in various fields of gaze.

myopia: condition of ametropia in which sharp images form anterior to the fovea, thus indicating presence of excess positive vergence (plus power) and requiring minus lenses for correction.

> *Axial:* myopia caused by longer-than-average globe length, measured from the pupil center to the retina.
>
> *Curvature:* myopia caused by less-than-average radius of curvature of the cornea, thus resulting in greater-than-average power measured in diopters.
>
> *Index:* myopia caused by an increase in the refractive index of the crystalline lens.

myopic shifts: changes in the refractive status of the eye that increase plus vergence (plus power), thus moving sharp images from the fovea to an anterior position and requiring minus lenses for correction.

N

nanometer: unit of measurement in the metric system [1 nm = 10^{-9} m = 10^{-7} cm = 10^{-6} mm].

Nd:YAG: laser using neodymium, yttrium, aluminum, and garnet as lasing media.

near point: in optics, the nearest point that is in focus, depending on the available accommodation.

nearsightedness: ability to see at near but not far away; a characteristic of myopia.

negative vergence: refers to the divergence of light rays.

nominal power: algebraic sum of the powers of the front (plus) and back (minus) surfaces of a spectacle lens. Does not account for the refractive index of the lens material.

normal: in optics, an imaginary line drawn at 90 degrees to a refracting or reflecting surface.

O

object distance: distance (in meters) of an object in front of a lens.

object-image relationships: comparison of sizes of objects and images to determine magnification.

object size: dimension of an object emitting incident light rays.

object vergence: divergence or convergence of incident rays (expressed in diopters), and obtained by the inverse (in meters) of the distance of an object from a lens.

objective findings: any finding that does not include response(s) from a patient.

occlusion therapy: management of amblyopia by practitioners. The better eye is typically occluded (or its image made blurry by instilling cycloplegic drops) in order to improve vision in the amblyopic eye.

ophthalmometer: generic name for an instrument for measuring corneal curvature in radius of curvature and diopters.

ophthalmoscope: instrument for viewing the interior of an eye. Two types: *direct*—instrument creates an upright image in a smaller field of view due to greater magnification (15x); *indirect*—instrument creates an inverted image in a larger field of view due to lesser magnification (5x).

optic axis: an imaginary line at 90 degrees to the center of a lens along which incident light rays are not refracted.

optical center (OC): the center of a lens through which the optic axis passes.

optical center (OC) displacement: distance from the OC to the pupil center.

optical cross: a pictorial representation of the power of a lens by using two meridians at 90 degrees to each other.

optical media: any transparent material through which light can pass. In the eye: tears, cornea, aqueous, lens, and vitreous.

orange: visible light in the electromagnetic spectrum whose wavelength is longer than green but shorter than red.

orange dye: see *fluorescein sodium.*

out of phase: wave propagation in which crests and troughs of waves do not travel together.

over minus: excessive minus, or inadequate plus, power in corrective lenses.

P

phacoemulsification: see *extracapsular cataract extraction (ECCE)*.

photoablation: use of light to change the radius of curvature and, thus, power of a curved surface, such as in refractive surgery.

photocoagulation: thermal destruction of tissues by lasers using argon or krypton as a lasing medium.

photodisruption: destroying the central portion of a posterior capsule opacity around the visual axis using Nd:YAG (neodymium, yttrium, aluminum, garnet) as lasing media.

photokeratoscope view: one of the views provided by computed corneal topography (CCT) in which Placido rings may be viewed in real time.

photon: a particle of light.

piggyback lenses: multiple lens system to correct a refractive error.

pinhole visual acuity: uncorrected or partly corrected vision produced by the central rays, which are present around the visual axis and, therefore, not refracted.

Placido disk: large circular disk with a central opening used to project and view concentric black and white rings in order to determine the state of corneal curvatures. Basis of computed corneal topography (CCT).

plane mirror: a mirror whose radius of curvature may be considered to be infinite and, therefore, without power.

plane surface: one of two surfaces of a cylindrical lens without power.

plano: no power.

plus cylinder form: system of denoting lens powers for correcting astigmatism using plus cylindrical lenses.

plus direction: more plus in plus lenses, or less plus in minus lenses.

plus lens: a refracting medium that provides positive vergence (convergence) and, thus, plus power.

plus power: positive vergence (convergence).

plus space: space behind a lens through which refracted light passes after being converged or diverged by a lens.

point focus: point at which refracted light rays come to a focus, producing a stigmatic image in plus spherical lenses, or point at which refracted light rays appear to diverge from in minus spherical lenses.

polarization: vibration of light in one direction.

population inversion: number of excited light particles exceeds the resting particles in a lasing medium.

positive vergence: plus vergence (convergence).

power of crystalline lens: average power in normal lenses is +19 D for distance. Near power varies depending on the available amplitude of accommodation (maximum of +14 D up to age 8, and decreasing to 0 D by age 72).

power of mirrors: reflecting power, in diopters, of concave and convex mirrors.

power meridian: curved surface of a cylindrical lens that provides all of the power.

Prentice's Rule: formula relating induced prism to the power of a lens and the displacement of the optical center of the lens away from the pupil center.

presbyopia: *presby* = old; *opia* = vision; condition of the gradual loss of accommodation with age.

Prince Rule: meter stick and Nearpoint Rotochart provided with refractors to measure ocular parameters at 16 and 28 inches (40 and 71 cm).

prism: wedge-shaped transparent medium whose refracting surfaces are at an angle to each other; *prism apex*—meeting point of the two refracting surfaces at an angle to each other;

prism base—wide part of the prism towards which refracted light rays bend and displace the real image.

prism diopters: see *prism power.*

prism images: real and virtual images produced by a prism. The real image is displaced toward the prism base, whereas the virtual image appears displaced toward the apex.

prism power: ability of a prism, measured in prism diopters (Δ or PD), to displace the real image toward the base of the prism.

prismatic effect: characteristics produced by spectacle lenses when the gaze is directed away from the optical centers of the lenses, and when the optical centers of the lenses are displaced away from the pupil centers.

PRK: photorefractive keratectomy; a surgical procedure to alter the curvature of the cornea and improve uncorrected vision.

pseudophakes: *pseudo* = false; *phak* = lens; refers to the presence of an IOL.

PTK: phototherapeutic keratectomy; a surgical procedure to decrease the irregularities of a cornea and improve the medical status of the eye.

pupillary distance (PD): the distance between the centers of the two pupils in binocular individuals. *Patient PD*—pupillary distance; *frame PD*—distance between the optical centers of the two spectacle lenses.

R

radius of curvature: radius of an imaginary circle produced when the profile of a refracting medium is extended to create a full circle. Term used for the cornea, mirrors, and spectacle, contact, and crystalline lenses.

rainbows: prismatic effect produced in the atmosphere by water droplets acting as prisms.

reading add: plus lens of a specific power used by presbyopes for magnifying fine print.

reading glasses: spectacle lenses that can be single vision, bifocal, trifocal, or progressive addition.

real image: in lenses, image produced in the plus space of a lens; in prisms, image produced by light refracted toward the prism base.

red: visible light in the electromagnetic spectrum whose wavelength is longer than blue, green, yellow, and orange.

red-free light: green light.

reflected light: light rays whose direction of travel is changed by a lens during total internal reflection, or by a mirror.

refracting device: a prism or lens.

refraction: in optics, bending of light by a transparent medium when incident rays strike its surface at an angle other than 90 degrees. Also refers to the medical decision making by a licensed practitioner to prescribe corrective lenses, which may not be performed by ophthalmic medical personnel.

refractive errors: myopia, hyperopia, and astigmatism, together constituting ametropia.

refractive index (RI): in any transparent medium, the RI is the ratio of the speed of light in a vacuum and its speed in the medium.

refractive surgery: surgical procedure to alter the curvature of the cornea and eliminate or reduce ametropia.

refractometry: measurement of refractive errors; may be performed by ophthalmic medical personnel.

Reichert Nearpoint Rotochart: meter stick and reading card provided with refractors to measure ocular parameters at 16 and 28 inches (40 and 71 cm).

retinal plane: an imaginary plane tangential to the curvature of the retina.

retinoscope collar: movable collar present on streak retinoscopes that can be moved vertically (downward in a Copeland; upward in a Welch-Allyn), providing plus power and enhancing the streak.

retinoscopy: process of viewing the retina and objectively measuring refractive errors.

ripple: waveform with crests and troughs.

risley prism: prisms mounted on each side of a refractor and used to measure horizontal, vertical, or compound phorias and tropias.

S

schematic reduced eye: system developed by Gullstrand and others to simplify optical characteristics of the eye, thus enabling easier calculations.

Seidel test: qualitative test to determine if a small incision on the cornea is sealed properly. Sterile fluorescein sodium is introduced on the wound. If it is not properly sealed, aqueous will leak, mix with the fluorescein, and appear as a green rivulet.

semicircular green mires: targets seen during Goldmann applanation tonometry, and produced when orange-colored fluorescein sodium is excited by blue light.

sharply focused streak: using a streak retinoscope to produce an enhanced (sharp) streak and estimate the amount of hyperopia.

Sin i: Sine (a trigonometrical function) of the angle of incidence, one of the variables in Snell's law.

Sin r: Sine (a trigonometrical function) of the angle of refraction, one of the variables in Snell's law.

slab-off: removing (slab off) a portion of the bifocal reading add to produce a prismatic effect and minimize image jump.

Snell's law: basic law in physics, light, optics, and ophthalmology, which states that "n_1 Sin i = n_2 Sin r."

Snellen eye chart mirrors: front surface mirrors used to project eye charts.

spectacle lens prism base: in plus lenses, the prism base is denoted by the optical center; in minus lenses, the prism base is denoted by the lens periphery.

spectrum: the sequence and range of visible and invisible electromagnetic waves.

speed: distance divided by time.

speed of light in a transparent medium: may be calculated by dividing the speed of light in a vacuum by the refractive index of the medium.

speed of light in a vacuum: 3×10^{10} cm per sec.

sphere power: the first value in a cylindrical and spherocylindrical lens prescription, and the only value in a spherical lens prescription.

spherical equivalent: dioptric value corresponding to the Circle of Least Confusion, and obtained by algebraically adding half of the cylinder value to the sphere value in cylindrical and spherocylindrical lens prescriptions.

spherical lens: lens that has the same power in all meridia (axes).

spherocylindrical lens: lens formed by combining a spherical lens with a cylindrical lens.

spontaneous emission: natural emission of energy by a substance.

squinting: decreasing the palpebral fissure to create a pinhole effect to improve visual acuity.

steeper cornea: a cornea with a relatively shorter radius of curvature and, thus, relatively greater power.

stereo Titmus test: ophthalmic test to quantify stereo vision in seconds of arc.

stigmatic: *stigma* = point; denoting the presence of a point focus, which is seen in spherical spectacle and contact lenses, and spherical corneas and crystalline lenses.

stigmatic ametropia: ametropia without astigmatism.

stigmatic image: denoting a point image formed by spherical spectacle and contact lenses, and spherical corneas and crystalline lenses.

stimulated emission: inducing a substance to emit energy; an important step in producing a laser beam.

streak retinoscope: a retinoscope whose filament and construction forms a longitudinal beam; common examples include Copeland and Welch-Allyn.

stroma: the thickest layer of the cornea.

subjective findings: data and quantifications based on responses by a patient.

synkinetic response (synkinetic reflex): accommodation accompanied by convergence and miosis.

T

the K: the lesser of the two keratometry readings used to determine the starting base curve for contact lens fitting.

tonometer: instrument for measuring intraocular pressure.

tools: metal blocks used by optical laboratories to generate the prescribed power on lens blanks.

total internal reflection (TIR): phenomenon when light is incident on a refractive interface at an angle of incidence greater than the critical angle for the material; in this case, none of the light is refracted, and all light is reflected back into the first medium.

toward the normal: bending of light during refraction.

transposing lens prescriptions: calculating the values of a lens prescription containing plus cylinder in order to derive the corresponding lens prescription containing minus cylinder, or vice versa.

trough: the lowest point in a wave.

true power: power of a lens that also includes refractive index of the material in addition to the powers of the front and back surfaces.

U

ultraviolet (UV): portion of the invisible electromagnetic spectrum whose frequency is greater than violet.

uncorrected refractive error: ametropia when corrective lenses are not in place.

unpolarized light: light that vibrates in all directions.

V

variables: values on both sides of an equation.

vergence: in optics, convergence (positive, or plus, vergence) and divergence (negative, or minus, vergence).

vergence equation: equation $(U + P = V)$ relating object vergence (U) and power of a lens (P) to image vergence (V).

vertex correction: adjusting the distance correction based on vertex distance.

vertex distance: the distance, in millimeters, between the anterior cornea and the back (D_2) surface of a spectacle lens.

vertically polarized glasses: prescription and non-prescription spectacle lenses used to block uncomfortable horizontally vibrating glare by only allowing vertically vibrating light to pass.

violet: visible light in the electromagnetic spectrum whose wavelength is shorter than indigo and blue.

virtual image: in lens, image formed in minus space; characteristic of minus lenses; in prism, image displaced toward the apex; in mirrors, image formed by convex and plane mirrors.

visual axis: imaginary line from an object to the fovea and passing slightly nasal to the center of the pupil.

W

wave: a ripple-like geometric form with crests and troughs.

wavefront: technique in refractive surgery to measure and decrease or eliminate high order aberrations, thus achieving "super" vision.

wavelength: the length of a wave measured from one crest to another, or one trough to another.

Welch-Allyn: a brand of streak retinoscope.

with motion: in lenses, the motion of the image movement observed as a minus lens is moved; in retinoscopy, the motion of the streak observed in an uncorrected hyperopic eye.

Worth 4-dot: subjective test to determine presence of fusion, suppression, alternating suppression, diplopia, and abnormal retinal correspondence.

Wratten filter: yellow filter used as a barrier filter to blue light when inserted in the path of reflected light from the cornea, while viewing green fluorescence used to evaluate the fit of a rigid contact lens in a slit lamp.

Y

yellow: visible light in the electromagnetic spectrum whose wavelength is longer than blue and green but shorter than red.

Z

Zeiss-Posner: a mirrored contact lens held against an anesthetized cornea for gonioscopy.

zonules: fibers attached to the ciliary processes and the equator of the crystalline lens capsule that support the lens.

Index

Printed in the United States
by Baker & Taylor Publisher Services